Workbook

Comprehensive Radiographic Pathology

Workbook

Comprehensive Radiographic Pathology

Fourth Edition

Ronald L. Eisenberg, MD, JD, FACR
Chairman of Imaging, Department of Radiology
Highland General Hospital
Oakland, California
Clinical Professor of Radiology
University of California at San Francisco and Davis
San Francisco, California

Nancy M. Johnson, BA, RT (R)(CV)(CT)(QM)
Faculty, Medical Radiography Program
GateWay Community College
Phoenix, Arizona

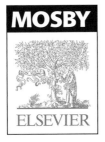

11830 Westline Industrial Drive
St. Louis, Missouri 63146

Workbook for Comprehensive Radiographic Pathology

ISBN-13: 978-0-323-04219-2
ISBN-10: 0-323-04219-8

ISBN-13: 978-0-323-04219-2
ISBN-10: 0-323-04219-8

Publisher: Jeanne Wilke
Managing Editor: Mindy Hutchinson
Associate Developmental Editor: Christina Pryor
Publishing Services Manager: Pat Joiner
Senior Project Manager: Rachel E. Dowell
Design Direction: Andrea Lutes

Printed in the United States of America

Last digit is the print number: 9 8 7 6 5 4 3 2 1

Contents

1 Introduction to Pathology, **1**
2 Specialized Imaging Techniques, **11**
3 Respiratory System, **19**
4 Skeletal System, **33**
5 Gastrointestinal System, **51**
6 Urinary System, **73**
7 Cardiovascular System, **89**
8 Nervous System, **107**
9 Hematopoietic System, **131**
10 Endocrine System, **141**
11 Reproductive System, **153**
12 Miscellaneous Diseases, **167**
Answer Key, **179**

1 Introduction to Pathology

OBJECTIVES

In addition to the objectives listed at the beginning of Chapter 1 in the textbook, the user should be able to:

1. Classify the more common disease categories described in this chapter.

   ✓ edema
   ✓ hemorrhage
   ✓ hereditary
   ✓ infarction
   ✓ iatrogenic
   ✓ idiopathic

   ✓ immunity
   ✓ inflammation
   ✓ ischemia
   ✓ neoplasia
   ✓ pathology

2. Define or describe the following terms from this chapter:

   ✓ abscess
   ✓ acquired immunodeficiency syndrome
   ✓ antibodies
   ✓ antigens
   ✓ aplasia
   ✓ atrophy
   ✓ bacteremia
   ✓ benign
   ✓ cancer
   ✓ dysplasia
   ✓ exudate
   ✓ grading
   ✓ granulomatous
   ✓ hematoma

   ✓ hyperemia
   ✓ hypertrophy
   ✓ hypoplasia
   ✓ malignant
   ✓ nosocomial
   ✓ permeable
   ✓ pyogenic
   ✓ scar
   ✓ seeding
   ✓ staging
   ✓ toxins
   ✓ transudate
   ✓ vaccine

EXERCISE 1—FILL IN THE BLANK

Complete the following questions by writing the correct term(s) in the blank(s) provided.

1. The study of diseases that can cause abnormalities in the structure or function of various organ systems is

   _____.

2. The measurable characteristics the patient exhibits as a result of the disease process are referred to as

   _____.

3. The characteristics that the patient feels and describes as their condition as a result of a disease process are

   _____.

4. Alterations of cell growth are known as _____.

5. Adverse patient conditions caused by physicians and their treatment are known as _____.

1

6. In some cases the underlying cause is unknown, and this type of disease is termed _____.

7. Infections contracted at a healthcare facility are _____ infections.

8. Contagious diseases contracted outside the healthcare facility are known as _____.

9. The immediate response the body tissue has to a local injury is _____.

10. As a result of inflammation, there are four overlapping responses, which are:

    a. _____

    b. _____

    c. _____

    d. _____

11. The term _____ indicates the ability of fluids to pass from one structure to another.

12. Inflammatory _____ causes the swelling associated with the inflammatory process caused by protein-rich fluid resulting in pressure and pain.

13. Fibrous scar tissue replaces destroyed tissue with _____ tissue.

14. Fibrous scars are a result of strong connective tissue contracting to form a(n) _____ in the abdomen.

15. A protruding tumorlike scar, a(n) _____, results from an accumulation of excessive amounts of collagen.

16. List the five clinical signs of acute inflammation.

    a. _____

    b. _____

    c. _____

    d. _____

    e. _____

17. Microcirculation at the injury site results in _____ and _____.

18. Swelling because of the exudate is also known as _____.

19. As a result of the swelling, the pressure on the nerve endings causes _____ and possible

    _____.

20. The presence of _____ bacteria leads to the production of pus containing dead white blood cells, inflammatory exudate, and bacteria.

21. The specific inflammation associated with pus formation is _____.

22. A(n) _____ is the result of a pyogenic infection encapsulating.

23. When a pyogenic microorganism invades the blood vessel, _____ may cause involvement of other organs or tissue in the body.

24. An abnormal accumulation of fluid in intercellular tissue spaces or body cavities is known as

_____.

25. The general accumulation of fluid throughout the body is _____.

26. When extravascular fluid accumulates in pleural or pericardial cavities, it is described by the term

_____.

27. When extravascular fluid accumulates in the abdominal cavity, it is described by the term

_____.

28. An interference of the blood supply possibly caused by arterial narrowing or disease is

_____.

29. Localized ischemic necrosis within a tissue or organ caused by vascular supply or drainage is caused by a(n)

_____.

30. Thrombosis or embolic occlusions cause almost all _____.

31. The implication of a ruptured blood vessel is _____.

32. When a blood vessel ruptures and accumulates within body tissue, it results in a(n)

_____.

33. A term that refers to the reduction of the size or number of cells in an organ or tissue is

_____.

34. The failure of normal development accounting for a small size is _____ or

_____.

35. When casted or immobilized, a limb may suffer a reduction of muscle mass, which is known as

_____ atrophy.

36. Loss of nerve function, hormonal stimulation, or blood supply causing permanent atrophy is also known as

_____.

37. Hypertrophy indicates an increase in the size of cells, whereas an increase in the number of cells is referred to as

_____.

38. A loss of uniformity of cells and their orientation, associated with prolonged irritation or inflammation, is

_____.

39. "New growth" infused with abnormal proliferation of cells that are out of control is known as

_____.

40. The study of neoplasms, also known as tumors, is _____.

41. Neoplastic growths closely resembling the cells of origin in structure and function are considered _____ tumors.

42. New growths invading and destroying adjacent structures that spread to distant sites are _____ neoplasms.

43. Malignant tumors are collectively known as _____.

44. Neoplasia consist of two basic components, which are the _____ and _____.

45. The name of a tumor is determined by the _____ tissue.

46. A benign tumor consisting of fibrous tissue is called a(n) _____.

47. Benign epithelial neoplasms with glandular characteristics are _____.

48. Malignant neoplasms of epithelial origin are called _____.

49. Adenocarcinoma refers to a malignancy of _____ tissue.

50. Malignant connective tissue neoplasms are _____, which tend to spread more rapidly than carcinomas.

51. Malignant neoplastic dissemination can occur by one of three pathways: _____, _____, and _____.

52. A tumor that penetrates the wall of the organ of origin and implants at distant sites is disseminated by _____.

53. _____ is assessing tumor aggressiveness (biologic behavior) or degree of malignancy, whereas _____ is the tumor extensiveness at the primary site and the presence or absence of metastases.

54. Diseases that pass from one generation to the next through genetic information are known as _____ diseases.

55. _____ genes always produce a particular trait and _____ genes manifest the particular trait when contributed by both parents.

56. When alterations occur in the DNA structure, _____ may result.

57. _____ react to foreign substances and bind to make antigens harmless.

58. Antibodies must have bound to antigens to develop _____.

59. _____ consist of dead or deactivated bacteria or viruses, whereas a(n) _____ is a chemically altered toxin.

60. An immune deficiency attributable to infection through retroviruses is known as _____

_____ _____ known to be caused by _____

_____ _____.

61. The viral infection most prevalent in inflammatory disease of the liver is _____.

62. Hepatitis _____ virus is contracted by exposure to contaminated blood or blood products, or through sexual contact.

EXERCISE 2—MATCHING

Match each of the following terms with the correct definition by placing the letter of the best answer in the space provided. Each question has only one correct answer. Please note that there are more terms than definitions.

1. _____ assessing the aggressiveness of a malignant tumor

2. _____ consists of a low dose of dead or deactivated bacteria or viruses

3. _____ coughing up blood

4. _____ critical reaction that can cause death

5. _____ difficulty in swallowing

6. _____ epithelial tumor that grows as a projecting mass arising on the skin or on a mucous membrane

7. _____ foreign substances produced by invading organisms

8. _____ large, cystic, benign tumor masses

9. _____ loss of appetite

10. _____ major metastatic route of carcinomas

11. _____ malignant neoplasms of epithelial cell origin

12. _____ malignant tumors from connective tissue, such as bone, muscle, and cartilage

13. _____ opportunistic infection

14. _____ refers to extensiveness of a tumor and whether or not it has metastasized

15. _____ soft fatty tumors

16. _____ tumor cells grow well; patient becomes weak and emaciated

17. _____ tumors composed of blood vessels

18. _____ tumors of muscle

19. _____ use of cytotoxic substances that kill neoplastic cells and may cause injury to normal cells

20. _____ without form (cells)

A. anaphylactic

B. anaplastic

C. angiomas

D. anorexia

E. antigen

F. benign

G. cachexia

H. carcinomas

I. chemotherapy

J. cystadenomas

K. dysphagia

L. edema

M. grading

N. hematoma

O. hemoptysis

P. lipomas

Q. lymphatic

R. myomas

S. *Pneumocystis carinii* pneumonia

T. polyp

U. sarcomas

V. staging

W. vaccine

5

Circle the best answer for the following multiple choice questions.

1. The study of diseases that can cause abnormalities in the structure or function of various organ systems is
   a. oncology
   b. physiology
   c. pathology
   d. biology

2. A disease with an unknown cause is referred to as
   a. iatrogenic
   b. idiopathic
   c. nosocomial
   d. community acquired

3. A low-protein fluid that builds up in the tissue such as seen in pulmonary edema is
   a. hyperemia
   b. exudate
   c. transudate
   d. phagocytosis

4. In cases of severe pulmonary edema, the technologist may find it necessary to change the technical factors by _____ the _____ to better illustrate the fluid.
   a. increasing; kV
   b. increasing; mAs
   c. decreasing; mAs
   d. decreasing; SID

5. The type of microorganism that leads to the production of thick, yellow fluid called pus, which contains dead white blood cells, inflammatory exudate, and bacteria is
   a. pyogenic bacteria
   b. a virus
   c. phagocytosis
   d. a fungus

6. A localized encapsulated collection of pus is called a(n)
   a. granuloma
   b. scar
   c. keloid
   d. abscess

7. An accumulation of abnormal amounts of fluid in the intercellular tissue spaces or body cavities is
   a. edema
   b. elephantiasis
   c. anasarca
   d. filariasis

8. A localized area of ischemic necrosis within a tissue or organ produced by occlusion of the arterial supply or venous drainage is
   a. a hematoma
   b. filariasis
   c. edema
   d. an infarct

9. A blood vessel rupture that is trapped within body tissue results in
   a. a hemorrhage
   b. a hematoma
   c. a hyperemia
   d. edema

10. What is indicated by an increase in the size of the cells in the tissue or organ in response to the body's demand for increased function?
    a. hyperplasia
    b. hypoplasia
    c. hypertrophy
    d. dysplasia

11. These make up the 44 chromosomes that contain thousands of genes with the exception of the X or Y chromosome.
    a. homozygous genes
    b. autosomes
    c. heterozygous genes
    d. variable expressivity genes

12. Dominant genes _____ produce an effect regardless of their homozygous or heterozygous status.
    a. always
    b. frequently
    c. infrequently
    d. never

13. An alteration in the DNA structure, a(n) _____, can be caused by radiation, chemicals, or viruses.
    a. gene
    b. expression
    c. mutation
    d. autosome

14. Foreign substances such as bacteria, viruses, fungi, and toxins are called
    a. antibodies
    b. immunoglobulins
    c. antigens
    d. histamines

15. A systemic disease commonly resulting from AIDS that characteristically affects the skin is
    a. *Pneumocystis carinii* pneumonia
    b. Kaposi's sarcoma
    c. hepatitis
    d. toxoplasmosis

SELF-TEST

Read each question carefully, then circle the best answer.

1. The body tissue's initial response to local injury is
   a. inflammation
   b. edema
   c. phagocytosis
   d. hemorrhage

2. The accumulation of abnormal amounts of fluid in the intercellular tissue is
   a. ischemia
   b. edema
   c. inflammation
   d. hemorrhage

3. Signs are
   a. what the patient feels
   b. characteristics that can be observed or measured
   c. the subjective symptoms the patient describes
   d. headaches and painful joints

4. The term used to describe the unknown cause of a disease process is
   a. iatrogenic
   b. community acquired
   c. nosocomial
   d. idiopathic

5. The interference of blood supply depriving organ cells and tissue of oxygen and nutrients is known as
   a. ischemia
   b. infarction
   c. anasarca
   d. filariasis

6. As a result of this process, a localized area of necrosis occurs within tissue or an organ, which is called
   a. ischemia
   b. infarction
   c. hemorrhage
   d. hypoplasia

7. What results in the accumulation of blood trapped within body tissue?
   a. hematoma
   b. hemorrhage
   c. infarction
   d. edema

7

8. An abnormal proliferation of cells outside the normal cell growth is known as
   a. cachexia
   b. cancer
   c. neoplasia
   d. sarcoma

9. If the genetic information contained in the nucleus of a cell causes abnormalities, it is considered
   a. an immunodeficiency disease
   b. an inflammatory disease
   c. a hereditary disease
   d. a neoplastic disease

10. Immunity can be attained by
    a. artificial means
    b. natural exposure
    c. vaccination
    d. all of the above

11. A disease process contracted in the healthcare facility is considered
    a. nosocomial
    b. idiopathic
    c. iatrogenic
    d. community acquired

12. Dysplasia is
    a. an increase in the size of cells
    b. an increase in the number of cells
    c. a loss of uniformity of individual cells
    d. a loss in the size and number of cells

13. There are four overlapping responses (blood flow, migration of white cells, digestion of dead cells and tissue, and repair) that cause
    a. edema
    b. inflammation
    c. hemorrhage
    d. infarction

14. Extravascular fluid in the lungs is known as
    a. pericardial effusion
    b. pulmonary effusion
    c. pulmonary edema
    d. hemothorax

15. An infarct can be caused by a thrombotic occlusion or a(n)
    a. hematoma
    b. hemorrhage
    c. granuloma
    d. embolism

16. Hemorrhage implies that a(n) _____ has occurred.
    a. interruption in the blood supply
    b. ischemic necrosis within tissue
    c. initial response to injury
    d. rupture of a blood vessel

17. In response to physiologic stimuli, cells may change in
    a. number
    b. size
    c. differentiation
    d. all of the above

18. Failure of cell development causes
    a. hyperplasia
    b. hypoplasia
    c. dysplasia
    d. neoplasia

19. Neoplasms that invade and destroy adjacent structures and spread to distant sites are
    a. benign tumors
    b. malignant tumors
    c. metastatic tumors
    d. fatty tumors

20. Determining the extensiveness of a tumor at its primary site and the presence or absence of metastasis refers to
    a. staging
    b. grading
    c. hematogenous spread
    d. lymphatic spread

21. Hereditary disorders that may not affect parents and only occur when a person is homozygous for the defective gene are
    a. autosomal dominant disorders
    b. dominant disorders
    c. mutation disorders
    d. autosomal recessive disorders

22. A type of artificial immunity that exposes a person to dead or deactivated bacteria or viruses is
    a. active immunity
    b. passive immunity
    c. community acquired immunity
    d. antigen immunity

23. HIV is the main cause of
    a. hepatitis C
    b. AIDS
    c. hepatitis A
    d. none of the above

24. The most common viral inflammatory disease of the liver is
    a. HIV
    b. AIDS
    c. toxoid exposure
    d. hepatitis

25. The form of hepatitis contracted by exposure to contaminated blood blood products, or through sexual contact is
    a. hepatitis A
    b. hepatitis B
    c. hepatitis C
    d. hepatitis E

9

2 Specialized Imaging Techniques

OBJECTIVES

In addition to the objectives listed at the beginning of Chapter 2 in the textbook, the user should be able to:

1. Describe briefly the theory of image production for the following specialties:
   - ✓ computed tomography (CT)
   - ✓ fusion imaging
   - ✓ magnetic resonance imaging (MRI)
   - ✓ nuclear medicine (NM)
   - ✓ positron emission tomography (PET)
   - ✓ ultrasound (US)
   - ✓ single-photon emission computed tomography (SPECT)

2. Classify the terms as related to specific imaging modalities.
   - ✓ anechoic
   - ✓ angiography
   - ✓ annihilation
   - ✓ attenuation
   - ✓ biologic/molecular map
   - ✓ CT number
   - ✓ diffusion imaging
   - ✓ direct fusion
   - ✓ echogenic
   - ✓ echo time (TE)
   - ✓ functional MR
   - ✓ gamma camera
   - ✓ gamma ray
   - ✓ helical or spiral scan
   - ✓ high signal intensity
   - ✓ hyperechoic
   - ✓ hypoechoic
   - ✓ increased uptake
   - ✓ integrated imaging
   - ✓ isoechoic
   - ✓ low signal intensity
   - ✓ multidetector scanning
   - ✓ physiologic map
   - ✓ positron
   - ✓ radiofrequency (RF)
   - ✓ radiopharmaceutical
   - ✓ repetition time (TR)
   - ✓ T-1/T-2 weighted image
   - ✓ tomography
   - ✓ volume-rendered imaging

EXERCISE 1—FILL IN THE BLANK

Complete the following questions by writing the correct term(s) in the blank(s) provided.

1. Beyond general radiography, the first new imaging modality was _____, which produced images without the use of ionizing radiation.

2. To visualize the fetus, today the safest modality is _____.

3. CAT stands for _____ _____ _____; today

   this modality is known as _____ _____.

4. The first alternative to image the brain was provided by _____

   _____, eventually replacing pneumoencephalography.

5. Scientists integrated strong magnets and radiofrequencies to develop _____

   _____ _____.

6. Researchers developed a positron-emitting radiopharmaceutical to produce molecular images creating the newest

   modality, _____ _____ _____.

7. The modality that combines digital images using hybrid equipment or special software is _____ imaging.

8. Sound waves produced by a transducer describe the imaging theory of _____.

9. Sound waves passing through water-tissue can produce reflections. These reflections are called _____.

10. In US, tissues transmitting sound waves easily are _____.

11. Strong reflections in US are called _____ or _____.

12. When two structures have the same echogenicity, the term _____ is used to describe the structures.

13. Doppler imaging is used to study _____ _____ _____ _____.

14. In Doppler imaging, color is used to represent the _____ of flow and _____.

15. Examples of acoustic barriers in US are _____ and _____.

16. Scanning using a narrow x-ray beam and computation of the attenuation coefficient, which is then displayed as a gray-scale on the monitor, is _____ _____.

17. The _____ _____ reflects the specific tissue attenuation as relative to water in CT.

18. The highest CT number represents _____ and is _____.

19. The areas that appear black on CT have a _____ CT number denoting _____.

20. High-resolution images indicate that the thin sections must be _____ mm or less.

21. Multiple single scan CT equipment has been replaced by _____ or _____ scanners.

22. The newest CT scanners have _____ to produce 4 to 64 slices per scan rotation.

23. Integrating all image data in CT by using software to produce 3-D images is _____ imaging.

24. To produce MR images, the technologist selects a pulse sequence, which includes the RF pulse and their timing usually represented by the _____ time and _____ time.

25. The most commonly used pulse sequence in MRI is referred to as _____.

26. Fat tissue, subacute hemorrhage, and highly proteinaceous material cause a high signal intensity appearing bright on MR _____ images.

27. Blood flow visualizes as a _____ on MR images, which contrast sharply with adjacent structures.

28. To better demonstrate the blood vessels _____ _____ is administered for MR angiography exams.

29. With the application of gradients, the random movement of water can be demonstrated in _____ imaging.

30. To ensure a greater contrast difference between fat and water, _____ imaging is used.

31. Injecting a radionuclide and detecting the gamma radiation describes _____ imaging.

32. The dose of _____ is calculated on the basis of the specific half-life and decay rate.

33. The decay of the radionuclide is detected for imaging purposes by a _____ camera.

34. An increase in uptake on an NM scan that is directly proportional to the emission of gamma radiation is known as a _____ _____.

35. To gather data from the three-dimensional perspective, the use of a rotating gamma camera is used in _____ _____ _____ _____.

36. SPECT imaging is useful in evaluating _____ disorders, infections, tumors, _____, and neurologic disorders, such as seizures and trauma.

37. The _____ for PET is different from that for NM and SPECT in that it decays by the emission of a _____.

38. The production of two high-energy photons in opposite directions is known as _____.

39. PET is especially useful for imaging in _____, _____, and neurology.

40. In fusion imaging, _____ imaging is accomplished with the use of software and _____ fusion imaging is a result of hybrid equipment.

Chapter 2 Specialized Imaging Techniques

Match each of the following terms with the correct definition by placing the letter of the best answer in the space provided. Each question has only one correct answer. Please note that there are more terms than definitions.

1. _____ a drug that emits radiation

2. _____ ability to combine images from different modalities into one image

3. _____ allows for faster imaging and easy reformatting in the coronal and sagittal planes in CT

4. _____ by using magnets and RFs, images with high soft tissue resolution are produced

5. _____ capable of producing images of the fetus without the use of ionizing radiation

6. _____ compiles images to provide a 3-D CT image, which is especially useful in visualizing the vascular system

7. _____ CT numbers represent this value

8. _____ equipment designed to integrate multimodality images

9. _____ gadolinium chelates are used to visualize the blood vessels

10. _____ has a gantry and x-ray tube, which rotates, producing cross-sectional images

11. _____ hot spots indicate an increase in uptake that is directly proportional to the emission of gamma radiation

12. _____ imaging especially useful in determining metastases in oncology patients to determine treatment

13. _____ in US, the term used when the organ tissues are very similar

14. _____ localizes the specific regions of neurologic function of the brain

15. _____ NM imaging with the addition of a rotating gamma camera

16. _____ on T1-weighted images, fat, subacute hemorrhage, and intravenous contrast material produce this signal

17. _____ the most common pulsing sequence(s) used in MRI today

18. _____ the radiopharmaceuticals are detected with this device

19. _____ the time between the end of the last RF pulse and the point when the receiving coil listens for the signal

20. _____ the value given to the amount of attenuation in CT

A. annihilation

B. attenuation

C. computed tomography (CT)

D. CT number

E. direct fusion

F. echo time (TE)

G. echogenic

H. functional MR

I. fusion imaging

J. gamma camera

K. gamma ray

L. helical or spiral scan

M. high signal intensity

N. hypoechoic

O. integrated imaging

P. isoechoic

Q. magnetic resonance imaging (MRI)

R. MR angiography

S. nuclear medicine (NM)

T. positron emission tomography (PET)

U. radiopharmaceutical

V. repetition time

W. single-photon emission computed tomography (SPECT)

X. T-1/T-2 weighted image

Y. ultrasound (US)

Z. volume-rendered imaging

Circle the best answer for the following multiple choice questions.

1. Air and bone are _____ in ultrasound.
   a. hyperechoic
   b. anechoic
   c. acoustic barriers
   d. isoechoic

2. Helical scanning uses
   a. conventional single-slice scans
   b. table movement during scanning
   c. continuous x-ray exposure during scanning
   d. b and c

3. Cross-sectional images produced by high frequency sound waves is the modality of
   a. US
   b. CT
   c. MRI
   d. SPECT

4. In US, the transducer
   a. records the changes in signal pitch and direction
   b. is made of tungsten
   c. produces high-frequency sound waves
   d. a and c

5. Tissue that is echo free or lacking in signal is
   a. anechoic
   b. echogenic
   c. hyperechoic
   d. isoechoic

6. The CT number represents the
   a. attenuation of specific tissue relative to water
   b. signal intensity
   c. tissue echogenicity
   d. radionuclide concentration

7. High-resolution CT
   a. requires a section thickness of 5 to 10 mm
   b. requires thin section slices of 1.5 to 2 mm
   c. decreases resolution
   d. increases volume artifact

8. The modality of choice for the spine and central nervous system is
   a. US
   b. CT
   c. MRI
   d. SPECT

9. The time it takes to play out the entire set of RF pulses before repeating is
   a. repetition time
   b. echo time
   c. RF pulsing
   d. a T1-weighted image

10. On MRI, blood flow is described as a
    a. signal void
    b. high signal intensity
    c. low signal intensity
    d. bright reflection

11. Tissue suppression in MRI
    a. creates a greater difference in tissue contrast
    b. is used in the neck, abdomen, and pelvis
    c. helps to differentiate tumor tissue when tissue is close in consistency
    d. all of the above

12. Molecular movement and random thermal motion are what _____ MR images rely on to produce an image.
    a. diffusion
    b. fat-suppressed
    c. functional
    d. spectroscopic

13. Gamma radiation detected by a gamma camera is emitted by
    a. gadolinium chelates
    b. iodinated contrast agents
    c. radiopharmaceuticals
    d. none of the above

14. In the gamma camera, when the gamma rays interact with the crystals, they produce
    a. electromagnetic frequencies
    b. light
    c. radiation
    d. sound waves

15. The advantage of NM is that
    a. a physiologic map is produced
    b. an anatomic map is produced
    c. earlier detection of a disease process is produced in comparison with plain radiographs
    d. more than one of the above, but not all
    e. all of the above

16. The major difference between SPECT and NM procedures is that
    a. NM produces a 3-D image, whereas SPECT does not
    b. SPECT cameras rotate independently around the patient, whereas the NM gamma camera is stationary
    c. NM uses radiopharmaceuticals that produce higher doses than those used in SPECT
    d. There are not any differences between NM scans and SPECT scans

17. In PET scanning, the radiopharmaceutical produces
    a. a neutron
    b. a positron
    c. an electron
    d. an x-ray

18. The modality that best demonstrates treatment results and is the most effective to illustrate recurring tumor growth is
    a. MRI
    b. SPECT
    c. NM
    d. PET

19. The modality that has been found to best demonstrate the physiologic changes in Alzheimer's disease is
    a. MRI
    b. SPECT
    c. CT
    d. PET

20. The imaging modality that best demonstrates molecular-physiologic and anatomic relationships is
    a. fusion imaging
    b. PET
    c. CT
    d. SPECT

SELF-TEST

Read each question carefully, then circle the best answer.

1. The modality to best demonstrate the fetus without the use of ionizing radiation is
    a. CT
    b. MRI
    c. NM
    d. US

2. Computed axial tomography provides a
    a. cross-sectional view of anatomy
    b. physiologic map
    c. molecular map
    d. superimposed image of anatomic structures

3. The modality that provides three-dimensional images (axial, coronal, and sagittal) using RF pulses is
    a. US
    b. CT
    c. MRI
    d. NM

4. Using a radiopharmaceutical, computer, and rotating gamma camera provided diagnosticians with
    a. a cross-sectional view of anatomy
    b. a three-dimensional physiologic map
    c. anterior and posterior nuclear medicine images
    d. a three-dimensional anatomic map

Chapter **2** **Specialized Imaging Techniques**

5. The development of a radiopharmaceutical emitting positrons and the ability of gamma camera movement resulted in
   a. CT
   b. SPECT
   c. PET
   d. MRI

6. Echoes received by the transducer are the result of interaction between
   a. sounds and tissue
   b. RFs and a magnet
   c. x-ray and detectors
   d. radionuclides and a gamma camera

7. Tissue that produces a relatively strong reflection (echo) and appears as a bright intensity is said to be
   a. anechoic
   b. hyperechoic
   c. hypoechoic
   d. isoechoic

8. The best and safest mode to visualize blood flow, direction, and velocity is
   a. US
   b. SonoCT real-time compound imaging
   c. MRI
   d. Doppler imaging

9. Radiographic differentiation of soft tissue using a narrow collimated x-ray beam is accomplished by
   a. MRI
   b. CT
   c. SPECT
   d. PET

10. The ability to differentiate tissue in CT is dependent upon the relative linear attenuation coefficient, which is referred to as
    a. the attenuation factor
    b. the calibration number
    c. the CT number
    d. echogenicity

11. CT scanning in a continuous mode using pitch variability
    a. is dependent upon multidetectors
    b. is dependent upon spiral or helical x-ray rotations and multidetectors
    c. indicates the use of conventional single slice scanning protocols
    d. provides subsecond scanning abilities
    e. b and d

12. The most commonly used pulse sequences in MRI are termed
    a. echo time
    b. RF pulses
    c. repetition time
    d. spin-echo

13. The T1-weighted image is dependent upon a
    a. short TE and short TR pulse sequence
    b. short TE and long TR pulse sequence
    c. long TE and short TR pulse sequence
    d. long TE and long TR pulse sequence

14. On T2-weighted images water appears
    a. as a high signal intensity
    b. as a low signal intensity
    c. as a dark region
    d. none of the above

15. MR angiography requires the use of
    a. a radionuclide to demonstrate the blood vessels
    b. gadolinium chelate administration
    c. iodinated contrast administration
    d. microbubble contrast administration

16. Signals radiating from the patient is how _____ images are created.
    a. CT
    b. NM
    c. MRI
    d. US

17. Radionuclides
    a. emit high frequency sound waves
    b. emit ionizing radiation
    c. produce complications similar to those caused by radiographic iodinated contrast agents
    d. produce pharmacologic side effects

18. The sodium iodide crystals detect _____ to create an image.
    a. gamma rays
    b. high-frequency radio waves
    c. high-frequency sound waves
    d. x-rays

19. The gamma camera contains _____ crystals, which produce light.
    a. meglumine iodine
    b. selenium
    c. silver halide
    d. sodium iodide

20. In SPECT, the device that detects the radiation emitted from the patient is the
    a. film
    b. gamma camera
    c. receiving coil
    d. transducer

3 Respiratory System

OBJECTIVES

In addition to the objectives listed at the beginning of Chapter 3 in the textbook, the user should be able to:

1. Identify anatomic structures on diagrams and radiographs of the respiratory system.
2. Describe the physiology of the respiratory system.
3. Differentiate the pathologic disorders of the respiratory system by defining the disease processes and their radiographic manifestations.
4. Determine changes in technical factors to obtain optimal-quality radiographs for patients with various underlying pathologic conditions.

Identify the anatomic structures indicated by writing the correct name in the space provided.
A, Structure of the respiratory system.

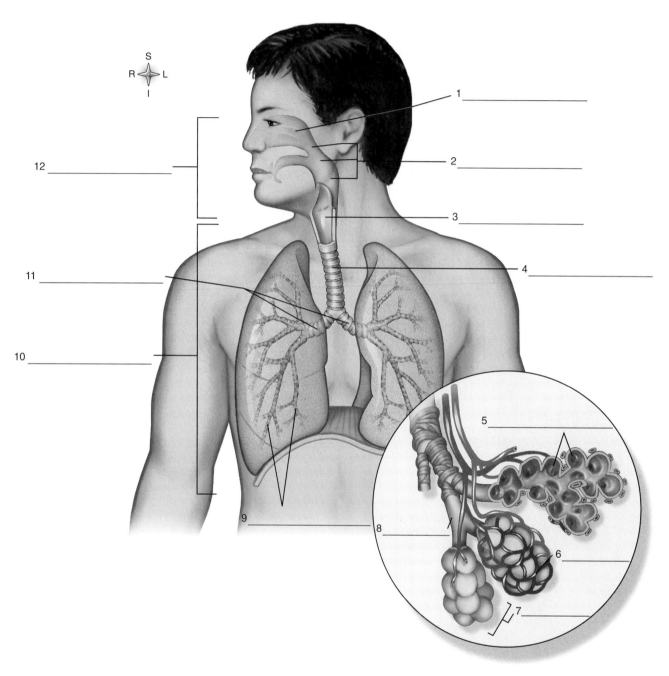

From Thibodeau GA, Patton KT: *Anatomy and physiology*, ed 6, St Louis, 2007, Mosby Elsevier.

Chapter **3 Respiratory System**

B, The lungs and pleura.

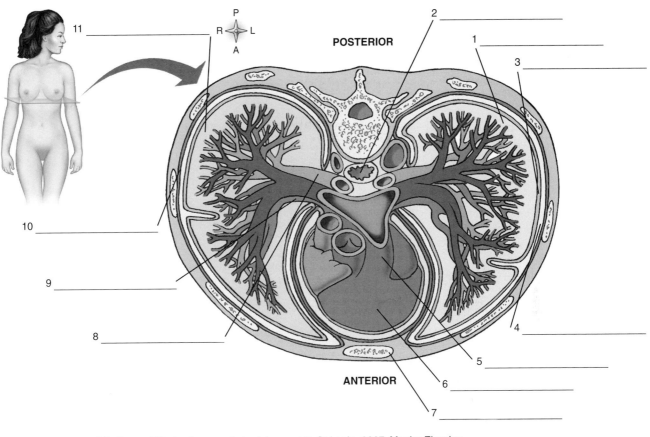

11 _____

P
R ✛ L
A

POSTERIOR

2 _____

1 _____

3 _____

10 _____

9 _____

8 _____

ANTERIOR

4 _____

5 _____

6 _____

7 _____

From Thibodeau GA, Patton KT: *Anatomy and physiology*, ed 6, St Louis, 2007, Mosby Elsevier.

EXERCISE 2—FILL IN THE BLANK: PHYSIOLOGY

Complete the following questions by writing the correct term(s) in the blank(s) provided.

1. The two major functions of the respiratory system are

   a. _____

   b. _____

2. The lower respiratory system consists of

   a. _____

   b. _____

   c. _____

3. The lower respiratory system is responsible for _____ from the upper respiratory system.

4. The tracheobronchial tree is lined with a _____ _____ .

5. The tracheobronchial tree contains _____ projections called cilia.

6. _____ prevent dust and foreign particles from reaching the lungs.

Chapter **3** **Respiratory System**

7. When cilia permits particles to enter the respiratory system (due to damage), the particles _____ to produce a disease process.

8. External respiration occurs in the _____.

9. Oxygen attaches to the _____ molecules in the red blood cells to circulate to various tissue throughout the body; this is considered _____ respiration.

10. The _____ and _____ muscles are stimulated to contract, causing the lungs to _____.

11. Pulmonary circulation provides the _____ with oxygenated blood.

12. The inner lining surrounding and attached to the lung wall is the _____ _____.

EXERCISE 3—FILL IN THE BLANK: RESPIRATORY PATHOLOGY

Complete the following questions by writing the correct term(s) in the blank(s) provided.

1. Irregular thickening of linear chest markings due to excessive viscous mucus is the radiographic appearance in

   _____ _____.

2. _____ consists of lipoproteins and provides the proper surface tension in the alveoli, allowing full external respirations.

3. _____ anteroposterior (AP) and lateral neck images best demonstrate a rounded thickening of the epiglottic shadow in this disorder.

4. _____ is characterized by the cause and location of the disease process in the lung.

5. A lung abscess appears as a _____ density characteristically having a

   _____ _____ _____ periphery.

6. A bacterium that is rod-shaped with a waxy coat allowing it to live outside the body for an extended time is

   _____ _____.

7. Pulmonary infiltration(s), most commonly in the periphery of the parenchyma, that may resemble pneumonia are

   the radiographic appearance of _____.

8. Respiratory syncytial virus is responsible for the increased rate of _____ infections because of the ability of the virus to persist on surfaces for many hours.

9. Emphysema, chronic bronchitis, and asthma are examples of _____

   _____.

10. In _____, the lung reacts to occupational exposure of silica, which results in extensive fibrosis.

11. _____ _____ causes peripheral atelectasis and pneumonitis due to bronchial obstruction.

12. An abnormal vascular communication between the pulmonary artery and pulmonary vein is a pulmonary

_____ _____.

EXERCISE 4—MATCHING: ANATOMY AND PHYSIOLOGY

Match each of the following terms with the correct definition by placing the letter of the best answer in the space provided. Each question has only one correct answer. Please note that there are more terms than definitions.

1. _____ breathing that supplies oxygen-rich air to the alveoli

2. _____ carbon dioxide regulates the respiration center in the brain

3. _____ cluster of alveoli

4. _____ consists of nasopharynx, oropharynx, and larynx

5. _____ extremely thin-walled sacs surrounded by blood capillaries

6. _____ fluid in the pleural space

7. _____ membrane attached to the inner chest wall (thoracic cavity)

8. _____ oxygen and carbon dioxide exchange due to cellular metabolism

9. _____ oxygenates blood and removes body waste such as carbon dioxide

10. _____ prevents dust and foreign particles from reaching the lungs

11. _____ provides the lung tissue with oxygen and nourishment

12. _____ respiratory muscles relaxing causes the lungs to expel air

A. acinus

B. bronchial circulation

C. cilia

D. expiration

E. external respiration

F. inspiration

G. internal respiration

H. lower respiratory system

I. medulla

J. mucous membrane

K. parenchyma

L. parietal pleura

M. pleural effusion

N. pulmonary circulation

O. pulmonary edema

P. upper respiratory system

Q. visceral pleura

Match each of the following terms with the correct definition by placing the letter of the best answer in the space provided. Each question has only one correct answer. Please note that there are more terms than definitions.

1. _____ abnormal communication between the pulmonary arteries and veins

2. _____ air-bronchogram is the radiographic appearance due to immature lung development

3. _____ arises from thrombi in the deep venous system

4. _____ condition of a collapsed lung

5. _____ consolidation of the lung parenchyma sometimes causing an air-bronchogram

6. _____ diseases caused by prolonged occupational exposure to irritating particulates causing interstitial inflammation

7. _____ fungal infection of the lung

8. _____ hereditary disease noted for secreting excessive viscous mucus by all endocrine glands

9. _____ most common type of lung cancer typically arising in the major bronchi

10. _____ necrotic area of pulmonary parenchyma containing purulent material

11. _____ neoplastic growth that is the result of an inflammatory process

12. _____ permanent irreversible obstructive and destructive changes in the acini

13. _____ primary carcinoma originating in the mucosa of the bronchial tree

14. _____ pus in the pleural cavity

15. _____ several conditions in which chronic obstruction of the airways leads to ineffective external respiration

16. _____ thin fibers embed in the lung, causing major fibrosis, and may result in mesothelioma

17. _____ this disease has four primary radiographic appearances: infiltrates, hilar enlargement, Ghon lesions, and pleural effusion

18. _____ viral inflammatory obstruction of the sub-glottic area of the trachea

19. _____ virus causing necrosis of the respiratory epithelium in the lower respiratory system

20. _____ widespread narrowing of airways caused by an increased response of the tracheobronchial tree to various allergens

A. asbestosis

B. asthma

C. atelectasis

D. benign granuloma

E. bronchial adenoma

F. bronchogenic carcinoma

G. chronic obstructive pulmonary disease

H. croup

I. cystic fibrosis

J. emphysema

K. empyema

L. hyaline membrane disease

M. lung abscess

N. pneumoconiosis

O. pneumonia

P. pulmonary arteriovenous fistula

Q. pulmonary emboli

R. pulmonary mycosis

S. respiratory syncytial virus

T. squamous carcinoma

U. tuberculosis

Circle the best answer for the following multiple choice questions.

1. To best demonstrate possible air-fluid levels in a lung abscess, the technologist should perform chest images with the patient
   a. upright
   b. semiupright
   c. recumbent
   d. supine

2. Croup and epiglottitis are best demonstrated on
   a. AP and lateral neck images
   b. soft tissue AP and lateral neck images
   c. increased kV AP and lateral neck images
   d. Posteroanterior (PA) and lateral upright chest images

3. Consolidation of the lung parenchyma most commonly due to a virus or mycoplasma is
   a. bronchopneumonia
   b. interstitial pneumonia
   c. alveolar pneumonia
   d. tuberculosis

4. Pulmonary mycosis is caused by a
   a. virus
   b. bacterium
   c. fungus
   d. parasite

5. Respiratory epithelial necrosis leading to bronchiolitis and resulting in interstitial pneumonia is
   a. alveolar pneumonia
   b. RSV
   c. tuberculosis
   d. bronchial emphysema

6. Large bullae develop, causing a reduction of the lung parenchyma due to alveolar destruction, which requires the technologist to _____ when the disease process is in its most advanced stages.
   a. increase mA
   b. decrease mA
   c. decrease kV
   d. decrease mA and kV

7. Extended occupational exposure to small particulates that embed in the lung parenchyma is
   a. pneumoconiosis
   b. pulmonary mycosis
   c. chronic obstructive pulmonary disease
   d. tuberculosis

8. Pulmonary metastases that typically appear as multiple round or oval nodules throughout the lungs is a
   a. miliary type
   b. hematogenous type
   c. bronchial adenoma
   d. granuloma

9. The modality that helps determine if a solitary nodule is benign is
   a. SPECT scan demonstrating a single hot spot
   b. PET scan detecting a single nodule with low cellular activity
   c. NM lung scan with decreased uptake in multiple lung segments
   d. CT scan demonstrating irregular spiculated lesion

10. CT demonstrates pulmonary emboli as a(n)
    a. filling defect
    b. contrast-enhanced region
    c. area of abnormal increased blood flow
    d. irregular nodule

EXERCISE 7—CASE STUDIES

The following are two case studies in which chest imaging was requested. After each scenario, you will see the image(s) and be asked to answer questions. Using the knowledge of imaging pathology, apply exposure factors and positioning criteria to answer the questions posed.

An adult male patient entered the healthcare facility with dyspnea. The following chest image was produced.

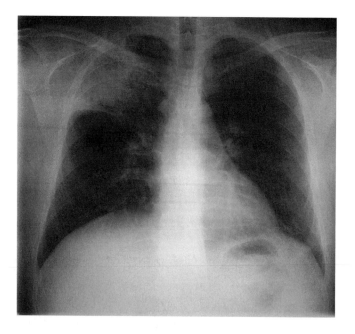

1. Is the chest image completed in the upright position as per routine chest protocol?

2. How is it determined that the chest x-ray is completed in the upright position?

3. Describe any subtle abnormalities seen.

4. Does the abnormality demonstrate air-fluid levels? If not, how would you describe it?

5. Were appropriate exposure factors used to demonstrate this pathologic condition?

6. As a radiographer, diagnosis is beyond the scope of practice; however, the radiographer should be able to recognize that the image demonstrates abnormalities. Any idea what disease process is being demonstrated?

CASE STUDY 2

An 8-year-old male patient entered the emergency room with a fever. The following PA and lateral chest images were produced.

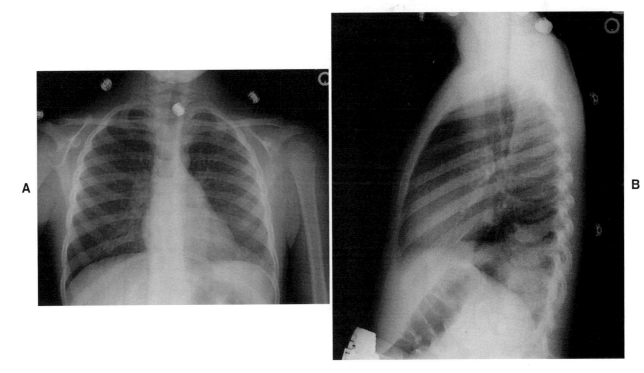

A

B

Courtesy Perry Trigg, Phoenix.

Images were exposed using normal technical factors. The radiologist's interpretation denotes mild infiltrates in the left lower lobe. Clinical correlation was recommended. The patient was given antibiotic treatment.

Chapter **3** **Respiratory System**

Seventeen days later, the young male reentered the emergency room with difficulty breathing. More upright PA and lateral chest images were completed.

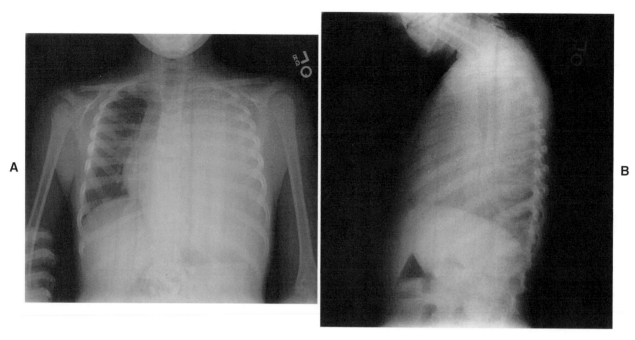

Courtesy Perry Trigg, Phoenix.

1. In the current chest image, are there differences from the initial image? How would you describe what is seen?

2. What positioning criteria must be followed to demonstrate a true mediastinal shift?

   Why?

3. How does the image demonstrate upright positioning and the use of a horizontal beam?

4. What other images could be completed that would demonstrate fluid movement?

Chapter 3 **Respiratory System**

In this case, what position would be most beneficial?

5. As a radiographer, diagnosis is beyond our scope of practice; however, you should be able to recognize that the image demonstrates abnormalities. Do you have any idea what disease process is being demonstrated?

SELF-TEST

Read each question carefully, then circle the best answer.

1. The major function of the respiratory system is to
   1) provide oxygen for the blood
   2) remove oxygen from the body tissue
   3) provide carbon dioxide to body tissue
   4) remove carbon dioxide from the blood
      a. 1 and 2
      b. 1 and 4
      c. 2 and 3
      d. 3 and 4

2. The lower respiratory system consists of the
   a. nasopharynx
   b. trachea
   c. oropharynx
   d. larynx

3. The gas exchange in the lung takes place in the
   a. bronchi
   b. bronchioles
   c. capillaries
   d. alveoli

4. On full inspiration, the diaphragm projects at the level of the
   a. 6th anterior intercostal space
   b. 8th posterior intercostal space
   c. 10th anterior intercostal space
   d. 10th posterior intercostal space

5. The disease process that is characterized by the secretion of excessive viscous mucus is
   a. cystic fibrosis
   b. tuberculosis
   c. hyaline membrane disease
   d. croup

6. Lack of lung development in premature infants that radiographically demonstrates as an air-bronchogram is
   a. cystic fibrosis
   b. tuberculosis
   c. hyaline membrane disease
   d. croup

7. Major radiographic signs are pulmonary overinflation, alterations in pulmonary vascularization, and bullae formation in
   a. chronic obstructive pulmonary disease
   b. emphysema
   c. asthma
   d. histoplasmosis

8. The most common work-related lung disease is
   a. silicosis
   b. anthracosis
   c. asbestosis
   d. pulmonary mycosis

9. Pneumoconiosis demonstrates radiographically as
   a. pleural effusion
   b. pulmonary edema
   c. scattered nodules and pleural thickening
   d. hemothorax

10. Granulomas represent
    a. benign lung tumors
    b. scarred lung tissue due to infection
    c. cancerous lung nodules
    d. metastatic pulmonary disease

11. Lung cancers originating in the glandular structures of the bronchial tree are known as
    a. bronchiolar carcinoma
    b. alveolar cell carcinoma
    c. bronchial adenoma
    d. bronchogenic carcinoma

12. A staphylococcal infection primarily in the bronchi or bronchiolar mucosa describes
    a. bronchopneumonia
    b. interstitial pneumonia
    c. aspiration pneumonia
    d. pulmonary mycosis

13. Pneumonia demonstrates radiographically as a(n)
    a. opacification
    b. radiolucency
    c. decreased attenuated region
    d. encapsulated area with an air-fluid level

14. Tuberculosis survives outside the host for a long period of time due to its
    a. shape
    b. waxy coat
    c. size
    d. droplet spread

15. A disease of the lung caused by a fungus is
    a. pulmonary mycosis
    b. pneumoconiosis
    c. respiratory syncytial virus
    d. chronic obstructive pulmonary disease

16. As a result of epithelial necrosis, the radiograph demonstrates an interstitial pneumonia in cases of
    a. respiratory syncytial virus
    b. chronic obstructive pulmonary disease
    c. pulmonary mycosis
    d. pneumoconiosis

17. If an upright image cannot be obtained, what other position would demonstrate pleural effusion?
    a. cross-table lateral
    b. lateral decubitus
    c. transthoracic
    d. Trendelenburg

18. Which of the following chest pathologies requires a decrease in technical factors from a "normal" chest radiograph?
    a. atelectasis
    b. pleural effusion
    c. pneumonia
    d. pneumothorax

19. Which of the following chest pathologies requires an increase in technical factors from a "normal" chest radiograph?
    a. atelectasis
    b. pulmonary edema
    c. pneumonia
    d. pneumothorax

20. Which of the following respiratory pathologies is not associated with chronic obstructive pulmonary disease?
    a. asthma
    b. bronchitis
    c. emphysema
    d. croup

21. Croup is
    a. a viral infection of the subglottis
    b. a thickened epiglottis
    c. a rounded thickening of the epiglottic shadow
    d. demonstrated best on a lateral soft tissue image

22. High-resolution CT has replaced V/Q scans in diagnosing
    a. pulmonary edema
    b. pulmonary effusion
    c. pulmonary emboli
    d. pulmonary mycosis

23. A filling defect seen in the pulmonary artery is indicative of
    a. pulmonary edema
    b. pulmonary effusion
    c. pulmonary emboli
    d. pulmonary mycosis

24. The abnormal connection between the pulmonary arteries and veins results in a pulmonary
    a. arteriovenous fistula
    b. effusion
    c. hemothorax
    d. embolism

25. The condition in which the lung collapses, causing reduced lung volume, is described as
    a. atelectasis
    b. pneumothorax
    c. hemothorax
    d. emphysema

26. Pneumothorax radiographically demonstrates as
    a. an area without pulmonary markings
    b. a fluid-filled pleura
    c. an air-fluid level in the lung parenchyma
    d. an enlarged heart

27. Thickened infected liquid or pus in the pleural space describes
    a. pleural effusion
    b. pleural edema
    c. empyema
    d. atelectasis

28. The mediastinum contains the following organs or structures:
    a. heart, great vessels, trachea, and thyroid gland
    b. heart, trachea, esophagus, and thyroid gland
    c. heart, mainstem bronchi, esophagus, and thymus gland
    d. heart, trachea, esophagus, and thymus gland

29. To best demonstrate the mediastinum, the chest image must be completed with
    a. no rotation, true PA positioning
    b. scapulas removed from the lung field
    c. AP since the mediastinal structures are located anteriorly
    d. none of the above

30. Paradoxical movement of the diaphragm best demonstrated on fluoroscopy describes
    a. eventration of the diaphragm
    b. elevation of the diaphragm
    c. paralysis of the diaphragm
    d. normal movement of the diaphragm

Skeletal System

OBJECTIVES

In addition to the objectives listed at the beginning of Chapter 4 in the textbook, the user should be able to:

1. Identify anatomic structures on diagrams and radiographs of the skeletal system.
2. Describe the physiology of the skeletal system.
3. Differentiate the pathologic disorders of the skeletal system by defining the disease processes and their radiographic manifestations.
4. Determine changes in technical factors to obtain optimal-quality radiographs for patients with various underlying pathologic conditions.

EXERCISE 1—LABELING: ANATOMY

Identify the anatomic structures indicated by writing the correct name in the space provided.
A, Long bone.

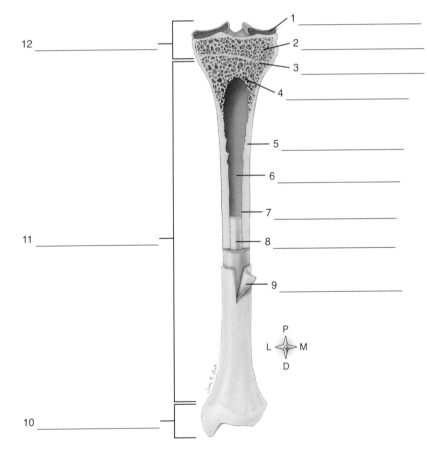

12 _____

1 _____

2 _____

3 _____

4 _____

5 _____

6 _____

7 _____

11 _____

8 _____

9 _____

10 _____

From Thibodeau GA, Patton KT: *Anatomy and physiology*, ed 6, St Louis, 2007, Mosby Elsevier.

B, Bone fracture and repair. Name the stages of trauma as related to the bone image.

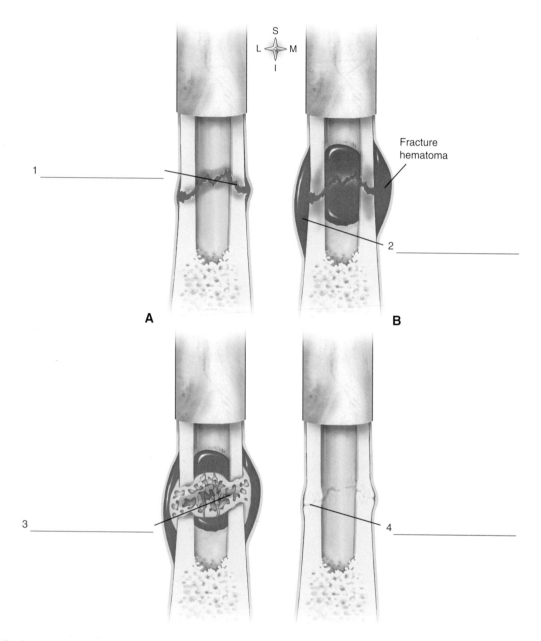

Fracture hematoma

1 _____

2 _____

A

B

3 _____

4 _____

From Thibodeau GA, Patton KT: *Anatomy and physiology*, ed 6, St Louis, 2007, Mosby Elsevier.

Name the stages of trauma as related to the bone image above.

A. Initial stage _____

B. Results in _____

C. New bone formation _____

D. Last stage _____

EXERCISE 2—FILL IN THE BLANK: PHYSIOLOGY

Complete the following questions by writing the correct term(s) in the blank(s) provided.

1. The two highly specialized connective tissues in the skeletal system are

   a. _____

   b. _____

2. The two major types of bone are

   a. _____

   b. _____

3. The two membranes associated with the bone are

   a. _____

   b. _____

4. The compact bone appears _____ and _____.

5. Weblike bone structure consisting of marrow-filled spaces is _____ or

   _____ bone.

6. Cancellous bone appears as _____ on the radiographic image.

7. Linear bone growth occurs at the _____ plate.

8. The two special types of bone cells are the _____ and _____.

9. The term for bone formation is _____ and the term for bone destruction is

   _____.

10. The skull and flat bones do not have a cartilaginous stage in bone formation so bone development occurs through

    _____ _____.

11. The diameter of the long bone expands or grows by _____ in the periosteum, producing new bone.

12. What five basic functions do bones perform?

    a. _____   d. _____

    b. _____   e. _____

    c. _____

EXERCISE 3—FILL IN THE BLANK: SKELETAL PATHOLOGY

Complete the following questions by writing the correct term(s) in the blank(s) provided.

1. A vertebra that has characteristics of the spinal column above and below is considered a

   _____ vertebra.

2. A splitting of the bony neural canal is referred to as _____.

3. The most common form of dwarfism is _____, which is the result of diminished proliferation of cartilage in the growth plate.

4. _____ is characterized pathologically by loss of joint cartilage and reactive new bone formation.

5. _____ is inflammation of the small fluid-filled sac located near the joint to reduce friction caused by movement.

6. A deep soft tissue swelling with obliteration or displacement of the fat pads and subtle metaphyseal lucencies describes _____.

7. Vitamin D deficiency in adults causes a loss of _____ as a result of the lack of calcium and phosphorus.

8. The most common metabolic disease of the skeletal system is _____ disease, which affects both osteoblasts and osteoclasts.

9. An _____ bone cyst contains numerous blood-filled arteriovenous communications.

10. The continuous external bridge of calcium deposit that extends across a fracture line is _____.

11. A fracture that may heal in a faulty position, resulting in impairment of function, is called _____.

12. _____ _____ is a chronic systemic disease of unknown cause, usually occurring in the small joints of the hands and feet.

EXERCISE 4—MATCHING: ANATOMY AND PHYSIOLOGY

Match each of the following terms with the correct definition by placing the letter of the best answer in the space provided. Each question has only one correct answer. Please note that there are more terms than definitions.

1. _____ bone formation from cartilage

2. _____ connective tissue bone formation

3. _____ dense structureless outer bone

4. _____ end of the shaft where the bone flares and becomes the epiphysis

5. _____ ends of long bones where growth occurs

6. _____ fibrous membrane covering the outer surface of bone

7. _____ flat bones ossify on their outer surfaces

8. _____ membrane that lines the medullary cavity

9. _____ portion of bone where blood production occurs

10. _____ resorbing bone cell enlarging the diameter of the medullary cavity

11. _____ shaftlike portion of bone

12. _____ trabeculae are contained here

A. appositional growth

B. compact bone

C. diaphysis

D. endosteum

E. epiphyseal cartilage

F. epiphysis

G. intramembranous ossification

H. medullary cavity

I. metaphysis

J. ossification

K. osteoblasts

L. osteoclasts

M. periosteum

N. resorption

O. spongy bone

P. trabeculae

Match each of the following terms with the correct definition by placing the letter of the best answer in the space provided. Each question has only one correct answer. Please note that there are more terms than definitions.

1. _____ "cotton wool" skull appearance

2. _____ a cleft in the pars interarticularis between the superior and inferior articular processes in the vertebra

3. _____ a deposit of uric acid in the joint

4. _____ a malignant tumor of cartilaginous origin that may originate anew or within a preexisting cartilaginous lesion

5. _____ abnormal decrease in bone density due to lack of calcium deposits

6. _____ arises in the bone marrow of long bones and affects young adults

7. _____ benign bone projection with a cartilaginous cap

8. _____ brittle bone disease

9. _____ caused by vitamin deficiency in children

10. _____ classic "sunburst" pattern with elevated periosteum

11. _____ degenerative arthritis

12. _____ failure of cartilage to form properly, resulting in dwarfism

13. _____ infection of the bone and its marrow

14. _____ inflammation of the fluid-filled sac usually due to repeated physical activity

15. _____ lack of neural tube closure

16. _____ marble bone disease

17. _____ most commonly affects the thoracic and lumbar spine with poorly marginated bone destruction often associated with an abscess

18. _____ proliferation of fibrous tissue in the medullary cavity

19. _____ rupture of central nucleus pulposus, most frequently L4-L5

20. _____ true fluid-filled area surrounded by a fibrous wall

A. achondroplasia

B. bursitis

C. chondrosarcoma

D. Ewing's sarcoma

E. fibrous dysplasia

F. gout

G. herniated intervertebral disk

H. hip dysplasia

I. osteoarthritis

J. osteochondroma

K. osteogenesis imperfecta

L. osteogenic sarcoma

M. osteomalacia

N. osteomyelitis

O. osteopetrosis

P. osteoporosis

Q. Paget's disease

R. Pott's disease

S. rheumatoid arthritis

T. rickets

U. spina bifida

V. spondylolisthesis

W. spondylolysis

X. unicameral bone cyst

Y. vertebral anomaly

EXERCISE 6—MATCHING: FRACTURE TERMS

Match each of the following terms with the correct definition by placing the letter of the best answer in the space provided. Each question has only one correct answer. Please note that there are more terms than definitions.

1. _____ bone response to repeated stresses

2. _____ composed of more than two fragments

3. _____ discontinuity between two or more fragments

4. _____ disruption of overlying skin

5. _____ encircles the bone shaft

6. _____ fracture healing process stops

7. _____ fragment torn from bony prominence

8. _____ incomplete fracture with the opposing cortex intact

9. _____ occurs at a right angle to the long axis of bone

10. _____ overlying skin is intact

11. _____ runs approximately 45 degrees to the bone shaft

12. _____ separation of bone fragments

A. avulsion

B. closed

C. comminuted

D. complete

E. displaced

F. fatigue

G. greenstick

H. malunion

I. nonunion

J. oblique

K. open

L. segmental

M. spiral

N. transverse

EXERCISE 7—MATCHING: TYPES OF FRACTURES

Match each of the following terms with the correct definition by placing the letter of the best answer in the space provided. Each question has only one correct answer. Please note that there are more terms than definitions.

1. _____ ankle dislocation with fractured malleoli

2. _____ avulsion fracture at the base of the fifth metatarsal

3. _____ avulsion fracture of the spinous process

4. _____ C2 fracture of the arch, usually associated with anterior subluxation of C2-C3

5. _____ comminuted fracture of the ring of the atlas

6. _____ isolated fracture of the ulna with associated dislocation of the radius in the elbow

7. _____ transverse fracture of the lumbar vertebra

8. _____ transverse fracture of the neck of the fifth metacarpal

9. _____ transverse fracture of the waist of this carpal bone

10. _____ transverse fracture through distal radius with dorsal angulation

A. boxer's

B. clay shoveler's

C. Colles'

D. hangman's

E. Jefferson's

F. Jones

G. Monteggia's

H. navicular

I. Pott's

J. seat belt

K. stress

L. torus

Circle the best answer for the following multiple choice questions.

1. The excessive proliferation of fibrous tissue in the medullary cavity describes
   a. achondroplasia
   b. fibrous dysplasia
   c. osteomalacia
   d. gout

2. The displacement of L4-L5 due to slippage of the inferior and superior intervertebral facets is
   a. spondylolysis
   b. spondylolisthesis
   c. a ruptured intervertebral disk
   d. a Jefferson fracture

3. A herniation of the meninges is
   a. a myelomeningocele
   b. a meningocele
   c. spina bifida occulta
   d. a Chiari II malformation

4. Bone that fails to resorb and causes a loss of bone marrow is referred to as
   a. osteomalacia
   b. osteoporosis
   c. osteopetrosis
   d. osteogenesis imperfecta

5. Severe osteoporosis and thin defective cortices resulting in multiple fractures occur in patients with
   a. osteomalacia
   b. osteoporosis
   c. osteopetrosis
   d. osteogenesis imperfecta

6. The hip may "pop" out of joint and a "click" may be felt or heard on clinical evaluation in children with
   a. chondromas
   b. herniated vertebral disks
   c. club feet
   d. congenital hip dysplasia

7. _____ may undergo spontaneous remission and has symmetric involvement.
   a. Osteoarthritis
   b. Rheumatoid arthritis
   c. Psoriatic arthritis
   d. Infectious arthritis

8. In _____, localized bone deficiency occurs as a result of decreased bone mass per unit volume.
   a. osteoporosis
   b. osteomalacia
   c. osteopetrosis
   d. osteomyelitis

9. After repeated attacks, the inflammatory reaction produces evidence of joint effusion and clumps of crystal urate in patients affected with
   a. gout
   b. osteoarthritis
   c. pyogenic arthritis
   d. osteomyelitis

10. Osteochondromas are
    a. dense round lesions usually in the outer skull table
    b. a growth parallel to the long axis of the bone
    c. usually found in the small bones of the hands and feet
    d. tumors that originate from osteoblastic cells in the bony cortices

11. A grade one spondylolisthesis is diagnosed when the
    a. sacrum is displaced forward
    b. fifth lumbar vertebra is displaced forward one fourth of the thickness of the sacrum
    c. sacrum is displaced completely posteriorly from the fifth lumbar vertebra
    d. fifth lumbar vertebra is displaced anteriorly three quarters of the thickness of the sacrum

12. In diagnosing spondylolysis, which additional projections will be most helpful?
    a. Standing AP and lateral lumbar spine projections
    b. oblique lumbar spine projections
    c. flexion and extension lateral lumbar spine projections
    d. standing flexion and extension lateral lumbar spine projections

40

The following case studies required skeletal imaging. After each scenario, the image(s) are presented and you will be asked to answer questions. Using the knowledge of imaging pathology, apply exposure factors and positioning criteria to answer the posed questions.

CASE STUDY 1

A patient enters the department with an order for bilateral hand images. The patient has stiff and painful joints. Anteroposterior (AP) bilateral hand images were taken.

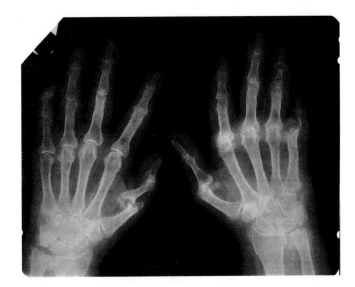

1. The interphalangeal joints should appear open on posteroanterior (PA) hand images. Name two positioning criteria to accomplish opening these joints.

2. Since the routine PA position is not evidenced, in this case what alternate projection(s) might better open the interphalangeal joints?

3. The joints appear to be enlarged due to effusion and misaligned. Name the category that this disease process is associated with: _____.

4. What is the differential diagnosis?

A young patient enters the radiography department with an order for bilateral lower leg images. The patient has had a low-grade fever and growing pains in the lower legs. AP and lateral lower leg images were produced. In this scenario, the right lower leg images were normal so only left lower leg images are included.

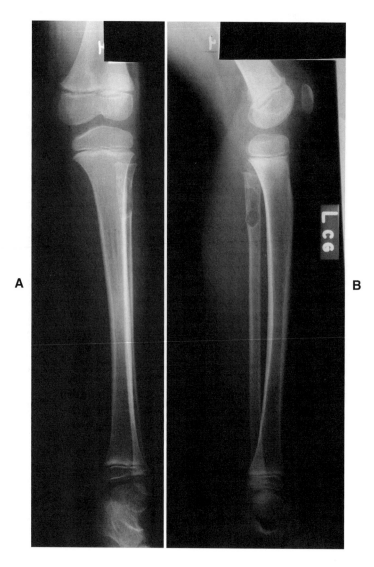

1. How does the lower leg image demonstrate that this patient is young?

2. What anatomic structure relationships indicate true AP positioning?

Is the lower leg in a true AP position?

If not, what positioning error has occurred?

3. Due to the AP positioning error, what pathology is difficult to visualize?

4. By producing a lateral image at a 90 degree perspective, what pathology becomes more easily identifiable?

5. Did the radiographer select the correct exposure factors to demonstrate the pathology in this case?

If not, how should the exposure factors be adjusted?

6. What could the lucency be the result of?

7. What is the differential diagnosis?

An adult male patient entered the emergency room limping. He came from playing basketball because he twisted his foot. A routine foot series was performed and is presented below.

A,B 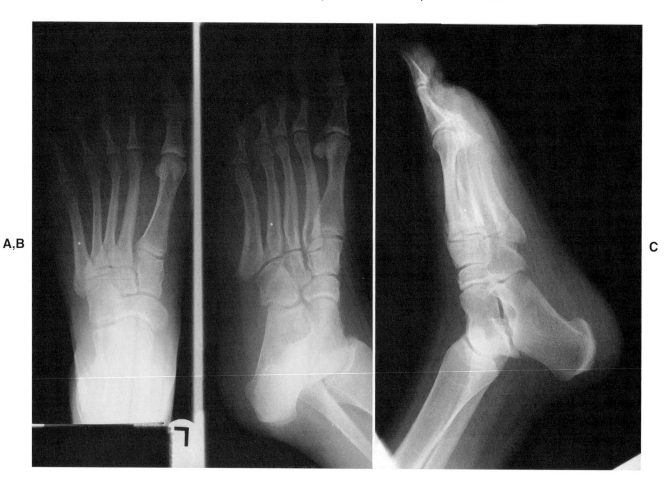 C

1. On the dorsoplantar projection, are any abnormalities noted?

   Describe what is visualized.

2. Are the toes properly exposed?

What changes could be made to better demonstrate the toes?

3. The oblique projection demonstrates an abnormality at the base of the fifth metatarsal. What is it?

4. On the lateral projection, is the area of interest well demonstrated?

What might the radiographer do to improve this image?

5. This image series demonstrates the importance of what positioning rule?

6. What is the most common fracture of the foot?

An adult male patient entered the emergency room by ambulance stretcher following a motor vehicle collision. The patient was in a cervical collar for immobilization purposes. A routine trauma C-spine series was performed. The resident and radiologist considered the images normal and "cleared" the patient. The patient was scheduled for direct coronal facial bones. The radiographer was uncomfortable in placing the patient into hyperextension without seeing the axial projections first. The following images were taken.

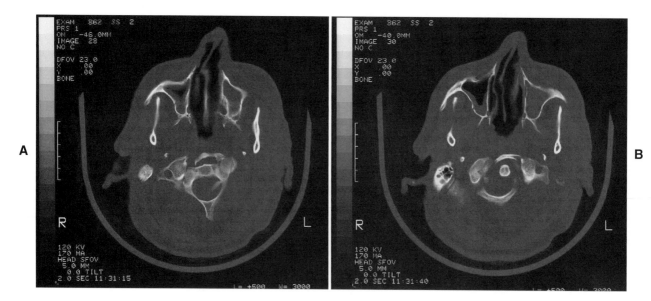

1. What structures demonstrate discontinuity?

   Which vertebra is fractured?

2. What is the name of this fracture?

3. By completing the axial projections first, did the radiographer practice outside his or her "scope of practice"?

4. If axial images were not ordered, can the radiographer add them to the scan series?

CT scans of the spine are becoming more common in trauma cases for just this type of situation. Scanners are much more efficient, provide multiplanar images, and usually take less time than the plain trauma C-spine series.

SELF-TEST

Read each question carefully, then circle the best answer.

1. For patients with severe osteoporosis, how should the exposure factors be adjusted?
   a. Increase kV and mA
   b. Decrease kV
   c. Decrease mA
   d. Decrease kV and mA

2. Osteopetrosis requires changes in the exposure factors. The radiographer should
   a. decrease SID
   b. increase kV
   c. increase mA
   d. increase mA and kV

3. The modality of choice to demonstrate cortical bone loss in osteoporosis is a(n)
   a. DEXA scan
   b. quantitative CT scan
   c. plain x-ray
   d. NM bone scan

4. The early stage of this disease process is seen as sharply demarcated radiolucency, which represents the destructive phase of
   a. Pott's disease
   b. Paget's disease
   c. gout
   d. osteomyelitis

5. Enchondromas are
   a. slow-growing benign cartilaginous tumors
   b. benign projections of bone with a cartilaginous cap
   c. eccentric lucent lesions in the metaphysis
   d. well-circumscribed extremely dense round lesions

6. An expansile lucent lesion with a thin sclerotic rim is a(n)
   a. osteoma
   b. bone island
   c. aneurysmal bone cyst
   d. unicameral bone cyst

7. _____ arise in the medullary cavity of the small bones of the hands and feet.
   a. Enchondromas
   b. Endodermomas
   c. Osteochondromas
   d. Osteosarcomas

8. For osteoid osteoma, _____ is used to best demonstrate the nidus.
   a. CT
   b. MRI
   c. US
   d. x-ray

9. The most sensitive imaging modality to demonstrate ischemic necrosis is
   a. CT
   b. NM
   c. MRI
   d. plain radiographs

10. Insufficient mineralization of the immature skeleton causing a cupped and frayed metaphysis in long bones is
    a. osteomalacia
    b. rickets
    c. osteoporosis
    d. Paget's disease

11. A "cotton wool" radiographic appearance is visualized in the reparative phase of
    a. Pott's disease
    b. Paget's disease
    c. multiple myeloma
    d. osteopetrosis

12. _____ is the least sensitive modality to demonstrate osteomyelitis due to its inability to demonstrate early destruction.
    a. X-ray
    b. CT
    c. MRI
    d. NM

13. Quantitative CT is one modality to demonstrate _____; however the DEXA scan causes less radiation exposure to the patient.
    a. osteopetrosis
    b. osteoporosis
    c. osteomalacia
    d. osteoma

14. The spine consists of an anterior and posterior column. When both columns are disrupted the injury is considered
    a. displaced
    b. stable
    c. undisplaced
    d. unstable

15. A transverse fracture at the base of the fifth metatarsal is called a _____ fracture.
    a. Jones
    b. Pott's
    c. boxer's
    d. Galeazzi's

16. It is common in a _____ fracture for the healing process to halt and the fragments to remain separate, creating a serious complication, possibly necrosis.
    a. navicular
    b. pathologic
    c. boxer's
    d. Jones

17. The malignant bone tumor most commonly found in the metaphysis of the knee is a(n)
    a. osteochondroma
    b. osteogenic sarcoma
    c. chondrosarcoma
    d. multiple myeloma

18. _____ causes destruction of the medullary cavity, producing an "onionskin" periosteal reaction.
    a. Ewing's sarcoma
    b. Osteosarcoma
    c. Chondrosarcoma
    d. Osteoid osteoma

19. To evaluate and grade spondylolisthesis, the radiologist needs a(n)
    a. standing AP lumbar spine
    b. oblique lumbar spine
    c. lateral lumbar spine
    d. standing lateral lumbar spine

20. To diagnose spondylolysis, the routine images should include
    a. AP and lateral cervical spine
    b. AP, oblique, and lateral cervical spine
    c. AP and lateral lumbar spine
    d. AP, oblique, and lateral lumbar spine

21. To best demonstrate a herniation of an intervertebral disk requires which of the following procedures?
    a. CT myelogram
    b. PET body scan
    c. US of the spinal cord
    d. NM bone scan

22. A transverse fracture of the spine often associated with significant visceral injuries is the _____ fracture.
    a. seat belt
    b. hangman's
    c. clay shoveler's
    d. Jefferson's

5 | Gastrointestinal System

OBJECTIVES

In addition to the objectives listed at the beginning of Chapter 5 in the textbook, the user should be able to:

1. Identify anatomic structures on diagrams and radiographs of the gastrointestinal system.
2. Describe the physiology of the gastrointestinal system.
3. Differentiate the pathologic disorders of the gastrointestinal system by defining the disease processes and their radiographic manifestations.
4. Determine changes in technical factors to obtain optimal-quality radiographs for patients with various underlying pathologic conditions.

EXERCISE 1—LABELING: ANATOMY

Identify the anatomic structures indicated by writing the correct name in the space provided.

A, Location of the digestive organs.

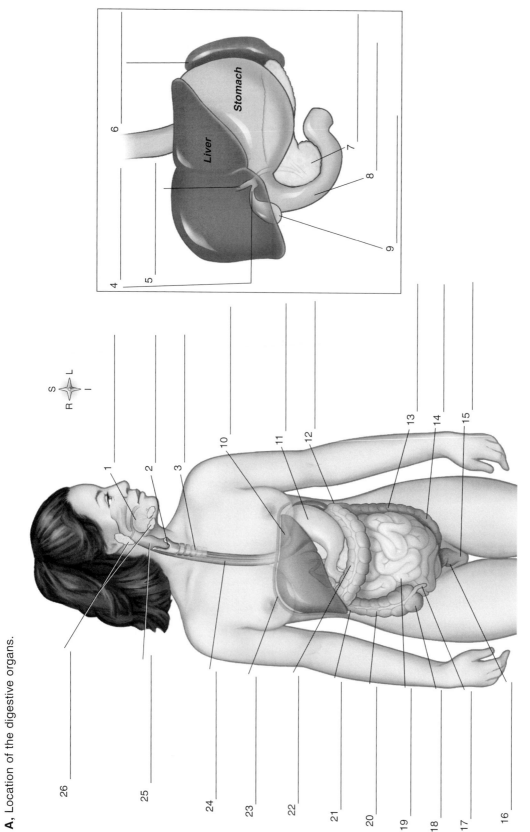

S
R ✦ L
I

Liver

Stomach

From Thibodeau GA, Patton KT: *Anatomy and physiology,* ed 6, St Louis, 2007, Mosby Elsevier.

B, Stomach.

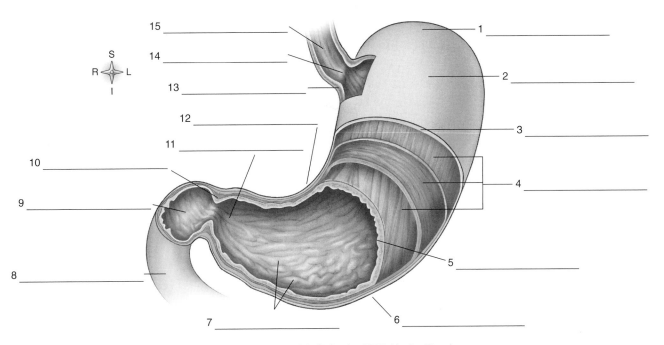

15 _____

14 _____

13 _____

12 _____

11 _____

10 _____

9 _____

8 _____

7 _____

1 _____

2 _____

3 _____

4 _____

5 _____

6 _____

C, Divisions of the large intestine.

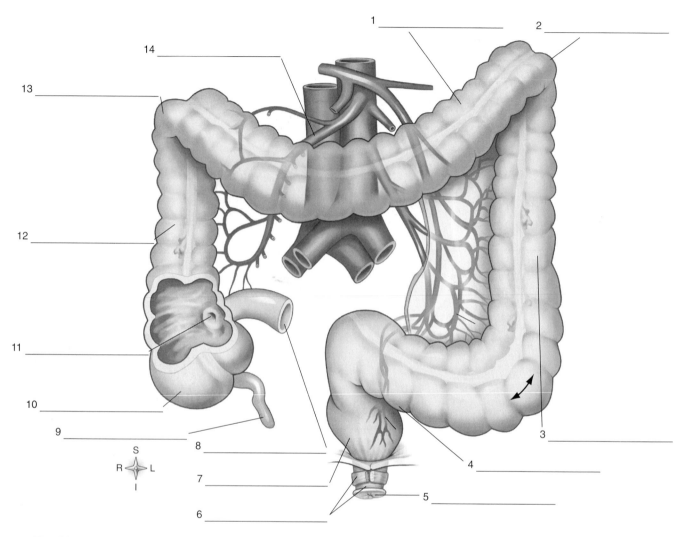

14

13

12

11

10

9

8

7

6

S
R ✦ L
I

1

2

3

4

5

From Mettler: *Essentials of radiology,* ed 2, 2004, Elsevier.

D, Ducts that carry bile from the liver and gallbladder.

10 _____

11 _____

9 _____

8 _____

7 _____

6 _____

5 _____

1 _____

2 _____

3 _____

4 _____

S
R ✧ L
I

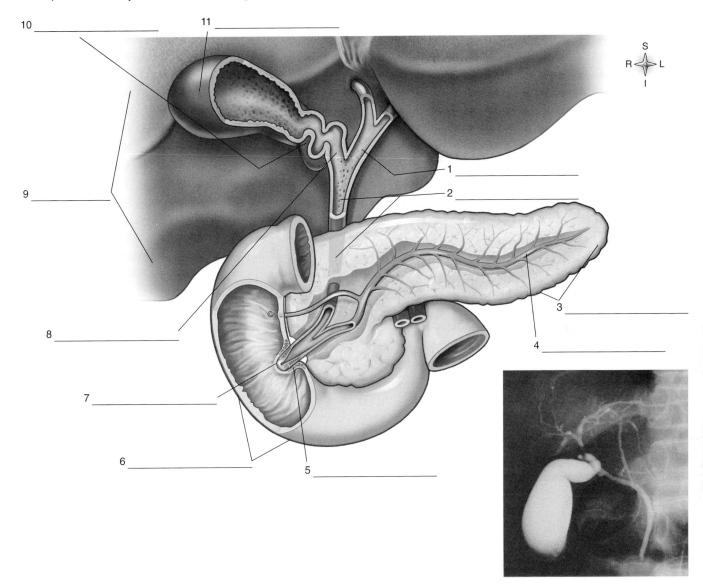

From Thibodeau GA, Patton KT: *Anatomy and physiology*, ed 6, St Louis, 2007, Mosby Elsevier.

EXERCISE 2—FILL IN THE BLANK: PHYSIOLOGY

Complete the following questions by writing the correct term(s) in the blank(s) provided.

1. The main function of the digestive system is to alter the _____ and _____ composition of food.

2. By altering the composition of food, it can be _____ and _____ by body cells.

3. The two types of glands associated with changing the composition of food are

    a. _____

    b. _____

4. Digestion begins in the _____ with _____.

5. Precise opening and closing of the esophageal sphincter requires coordination of many muscles for _____ to occur.

6. Acids and enzymes mix with gastric content, resulting in a milky-white _____.

7. Smooth muscle contractions that propel the gastric content through the digestive system are known as _____.

8. Fat digestion requires _____ to permit it to mix with water.

9. The pancreas produces enzymes for digestion of _____.

10. The completion of digestion means that the body can absorb nutrients through the _____ _____.

11. Four examples of fat-soluble vitamins are:

    a. _____

    b. _____

    c. _____

    d. _____

12. The pancreas secretes _____ and _____ to control the level of glucose in the circulating blood.

EXERCISE 3—FILL IN THE BLANK: GASTROINTESTINAL PATHOLOGY

Complete the following questions by writing the correct term(s) in the blank(s) provided.

1. In some cases of _____ _____, the upper and lower segments of the esophagus are blind pouches.

2. Double-contrast studies best demonstrate the superficial ulceration or erosions in the distal esophagus as streaks or dots of barium in _____ _____ disease.

3. Ingestion of _____ _____ produces acute inflammatory changes of superficial to deep ulcerations.

4. _____ diverticula arise from the posterior wall of the upper esophagus, sometimes large enough to almost occlude the lumen.

5. The radiographic appearance of esophageal _____ is serpiginous thickening of folds resembling the beads of a rosary.

6. Free air in the mediastinum or periesophageal soft tissue on radiographs implies a possible

_____ of the esophagus.

7. Irritants in the stomach, such as alcohol, corrosive agents, and infection, cause _____.

8. The enzyme _____ causes an inflammatory process to occur most often in the lesser

curvature of the stomach, resulting in a(n) _____.

9. _____ disease of the small bowel usually involves the terminal ileum and is a granulomatous inflammatory process.

10. In a _____ obstruction, a "string-of-beads" sign appears on upright abdominal images.

11. The small and large bowel appear uniformly dilated with no demonstrable point of obstruction on the abdominal

radiographs in a patient with a(n) _____ _____.

12. An appendicolith may cause gangrene or perforation, resulting in _____.

13. Patients with ulcerative colitis are 10 times more frequently affected by _____ of the colon.

14. A loss of haustral markings and deep ulcers outlined by intraluminal gas may indicate _____

_____.

15. A sessile polyp demonstrating growth with an irregular or lobulated surface on sequential examinations is

indicative of _____ _____.

16. Inflammation of the gallbladder, usually after obstruction of the cystic duct by a gallstone, is

_____ _____.

17. Calcification of the wall of the gallbladder is referred to as a _____ gallbladder, indicating

the possibility of _____.

18. Diffuse or focal enlargement of the gland with obscured soft tissue on _____ images is acute pancreatitis.

19. Pancreatic calcifications are the _____ finding in chronic pancreatitis.

20. The most common cause of pneumoperitoneum is associated with _____ of an

_____.

Chapter **5** **Gastrointestinal System**

Match each of the following terms with the correct definition by placing the letter of the best answer in the space provided. Each question has only one correct answer. Please note that there are more terms than definitions.

1. _____ bile is an example

2. _____ chewing

3. _____ consists of salts, cholesterol, and bilirubin

4. _____ excess glucose stored in the body

5. _____ fingerlike projections in the small bowel

6. _____ helps move the chyme through the digestive tract

7. _____ milky-white product found in the stomach

8. _____ produces an emulsifier

9. _____ produces enzymes to aid in digestion of proteins

10. _____ produces hydrochloric acid and proteolytic enzyme pepsin

11. _____ stores bile for use by the digestive system

12. _____ swallowing

A. bile

B. chyme

C. constipation

D. deglutition

E. diarrhea

F. emulsifier

G. gallbladder

H. glycogen

I. liver

J. mastication

K. pancreas

L. peristalsis

M. stomach

N. villi

Match each of the following terms with the correct definition by placing the letter of the best answer in the space provided. Each question has only one correct answer. Please note that there are more terms than definitions.

1. _____ any symptomatic condition or structural changes due to reflux of stomach content into the esophagus

2. _____ complete rupture of the esophageal wall

3. _____ dilated veins in the esophageal wall

4. _____ disease appears as a persistent collection of barium surrounded by a halo of edema

5. _____ esophageal lumen does not develop separately from the trachea

6. _____ fungus or virus causing a cobblestone pattern caused by deep ulcerations and sloughing of the mucosa

7. _____ incomplete relaxation of the lower esophageal sphincter causing esophageal dilatation

8. _____ inflammation of the stomach presenting as an abnormal surface pattern in the gastric mucosa

9. _____ inflammatory process of the stomach and duodenum caused by the action of acid

10. _____ most common manifestation of peptic ulcer disease

11. _____ most occur in the distal stomach and are of glandular origin

12. _____ most often this tumor is of squamous cell type and occurs at the esophagogastric junction

13. _____ much of the stomach lies within the thoracic cavity

14. _____ normal squamous lining is destroyed and replaced with columnar epithelium

15. _____ outpouching herniating through the muscular layer of the esophagus

16. _____ severe mucosal atrophy causing thinning or an absence of mucosal folds

A. achalasia

B. acute gastritis

C. Barrett's esophagus

D. chronic atrophic gastritis

E. diverticula

F. duodenal ulcer

G. esophageal carcinoma

H. esophageal varices

I. foreign bodies

J. gastric ulcer

K. gastroesophageal reflux disease (GERD)

L. hiatal hernia

M. infectious esophagitis

N. peptic ulcer

O. perforation

P. stomach cancer

Q. tracheoesophageal fistula

Match each of the following terms with the correct definition by placing the letter of the best answer in the space provided. Each question has only one correct answer. Please note that there are more terms than definitions.

1. _____ an inflammatory process usually of the proximal colon involving multiple noncontiguous segments (skip lesions)

2. _____ caused by previous surgery, peritonitis, or external hernias

3. _____ chronic granulomatous inflammatory disorder of unknown cause

4. _____ disorder of intestinal motility in which fluid and gas do not progress normally

5. _____ most common cause of bowel obstruction in children caused by the bowel telescoping into itself

6. _____ necrosing inflammation in the outpouches representing acquired herniation

7. _____ neoplastic growth with about half of the occurrences in the rectum and sigmoid most often in older men

8. _____ one of two inflammatory processes of unknown cause that primarily affects young adults

9. _____ outpouching representing acquired herniations of mucosa and submucosa through weak points in the muscular layer

10. _____ perforation permitting fecal material to enter the peritoneum, causing general peritonitis if not treated

11. _____ several conditions altering intestinal motility, usually functional disorders causing constipation or diarrhea (spastic colitis)

12. _____ twisting of the bowel on itself leading to intestinal obstruction

A. adynamic ileus

B. appendicitis

C. carcinoma of the small bowel

D. Crohn's colitis

E. Crohn's disease

F. colonic carcinoma

G. diverticulitis

H. diverticulosis

I. intussusception

J. irritable bowel syndrome

K. ischemic colitis

L. mechanical bowel obstruction

M. polyps

N. small bowel obstruction

O. ulcerative colitis

P. volvulus

Match each of the following terms with the correct definition by placing the letter of the best answer in the space provided. Each question has only one correct answer. Please note that there are more terms than definitions.

1. _____ cholesterol and pigment stones

2. _____ chronic process of destruction of liver cells and structure causing end-stage liver disease

3. _____ extensive calcification in the wall of the gallbladder

4. _____ gas-forming organisms that are facilitated by stasis and ischemia due to cystic duct obstruction

5. _____ loculated fluid collections resulting from the process associated with acute pancreatitis

6. _____ most common neoplastic process involving the liver

7. _____ neoplastic process occurring commonly in the head, causing the gland to have an irregular contour and semisolid pattern on the sonogram

8. _____ primary liver cancer

9. _____ protein- and lipid-digesting enzymes become activated within the pancreas, causing the organ to ingest itself

10. _____ sudden attack of inflammation of the gallbladder

A. acute cholecystitis

B. acute pancreatitis

C. cholelithiasis

D. chronic pancreatitis

E. cirrhosis

F. emphysematous cholecystitis

G. hepatic metastasis

H. hepatitis

I. hepatocellular carcinoma

J. pancreatic adenocarcinoma

K. porcelain gallbladder

L. pseudocyst

Circle the best answer for the following multiple choice questions.

1. In type II tracheoesophageal fistulas, the upper segment _____ and the lower segment _____.
   a. ends in a blind pouch; ends in a blind pouch
   b. communicates with the trachea; ends in a blind pouch
   c. ends in a blind pouch; attaches to the trachea
   d. ends in a blind pouch; ends in a blind pouch with both connecting to the trachea

2. The condition related to severe reflux esophagitis in which the normal squamous lining of the lower esophagus is destroyed and replaced with columnar epithelium is known as
   a. Barrett's esophagus
   b. esophageal cancer
   c. esophagitis
   d. gastroesophageal reflux

3. Mucosal and intramural inflammation of acute esophagitis may lead to pronounced fibrosis and stricture formation due to
   a. the ingestion of corrosive agents
   b. a herpes virus
   c. a fungal infection
   d. a polypoid mass

4. Irregularity of the esophageal wall indicating mucosal destruction possibly encircling the lumen is the radiographic appearance of
   a. gastroesophageal reflux
   b. esophagitis
   c. Barrett's esophagus
   d. esophageal cancer

5. The esophagus and stomach are distinguished by the difference in the mucosal folds; demonstration of the stomach in the thoracic cavity is a case of
   a. Barrett's esophagus
   b. esophagitis
   c. gastric reflux
   d. hiatal hernia

6. A functional obstruction of the distal esophagus due to incomplete relaxation of the lower esophageal sphincter is
   a. achalasia
   b. Barrett's disease
   c. hiatal hernia
   d. due to ingestion of corrosive agents

7. Nonerosive or _____ gastritis refers to mucosal atrophy causing a thinning and absence of mucosal folds in the stomach.
   a. alcoholic
   b. bacterial
   c. chronic
   d. corrosive

8. The radiographic appearance of an ulcer causes
   a. a bald appearance due to the lack of mucosal folds
   b. thickened gastric walls causing a stricture
   c. a rounded or linear collection of contrast surrounded by lucent folds
   d. infiltration of the gastric wall producing diffuse thickening, narrowing, and stomach wall fixation

9. To demonstrate air-fluid levels in the abdomen, the technologist will use
   a. a horizontal beam on the upright image
   b. a perpendicular beam on the lateral decubitus image
   c. a perpendicular beam to the semierect patient
   d. either a or b

10. The loss of motility in the small bowel is referred to as
    a. adynamic ileus
    b. mechanical bowel obstruction
    c. intussusception
    d. herniation

11. A "donut-shaped" lesion on a transverse sonogram of the intestine is suspicious of a(n)
    a. hernia
    b. intussusception
    c. volvulus
    d. adynamic ileus

12. In diverticulosis, the diverticula appear radiographically as
    a. round or oval outpouchings beyond the confines of the lumen
    b. round or oval outpouchings with extravasation indicating perforation
    c. inward extensions of the mucosal wall
    d. deep ulcers outlined by intraluminal gas

13. Discrete erosions appearing as punctate collections with a surrounding thin halo of edema are the earliest radiographic findings in
    a. colon cancer
    b. Crohn's colitis
    c. diverticulitis
    d. ulcerative colitis

14. Fine superficial ulcerations caused by inflammatory edema of the mucosa are indicative of
    a. Crohn's colitis
    b. diverticulitis
    c. ulcerative colitis
    d. ischemic colitis

15. The pathognomonic sign of a kidney-shaped mass (twisted bowel) with a thickened and twisted mesentery is suspicious of being a
    a. colon cancer
    b. cecal volvulus
    c. sigmoid volvulus
    d. hemorrhoid

16. The modality of choice to demonstrate gallstones is
    a. US
    b. CT
    c. MRI
    d. Kidney-ureter-bladder (KUB)

17. Large amounts of fat in the liver seen on CT or US images are suggestive of
    a. cirrhosis
    b. hepatocellular carcinoma
    c. hepatic metastasis
    d. an overweight patient

18. On US, an echo-free cystic structure with a sharp posterior wall and echogenic areas representing septations suggest a(n)
    a. pancreatic carcinoma
    b. chronic pancreatitis
    c. acute pancreatitis
    d. pancreatic pseudocyst

19. Gas appearing as a sickle-shaped lucency on an abdominal image requires upright patient positioning and a horizontal beam. If the patient is unable to stand, the technologist should complete a(n)
    a. right lateral decubitus
    b. left lateral decubitus
    c. semiupright KUB with the beam perpendicular to the patient
    d. KUB

20. CT best demonstrates blunt abdominal trauma for splenic laceration (the hematoma) as
    a. a crescentic collection
    b. focal enlargement
    c. a sickle-shaped lucency
    d. splenomegaly

EXERCISE 9—CASE STUDIES

The following case studies required imaging of the gastrointestinal system. After each scenario, the image(s) are presented and you will be asked to answer questions. Using the knowledge of imaging pathology, apply exposure factors and positioning criteria to answer the questions posed.

A 2-day-old infant arrives in the radiology department for an esophagram. The infant is not thriving and has not fed since birth. The following anteroposterior and lateral images were produced as part of the fluoroscopic procedure.

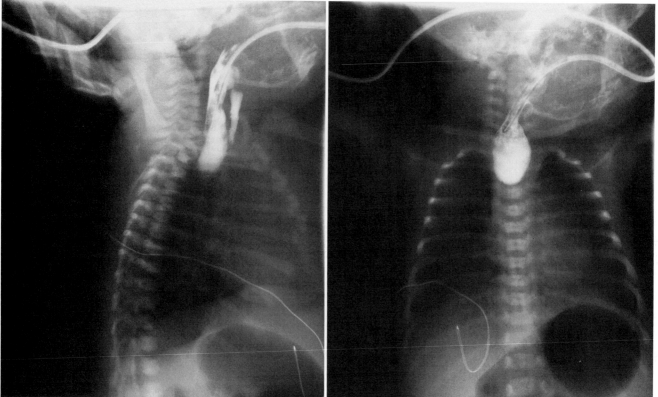

A

B

Courtesy Eric Bowlus, RT(R), Phoenix.

1. Does the technologist have the parents assist during the fluoroscopic procedure?

2. Barium sulfate is the contrast medium of choice. How does the radiographer prepare this agent?

3. On the image, what device is being used to inject the contrast agent?

4. The contrast agent is filling what anatomic structure?

5. What esophageal disorder are the images demonstrating?

CASE STUDY 2

A 46-year-old patient enters the radiography department with an order for a small bowel series. The patient is experiencing abdominal cramping. A small bowel follow through was done with images presented below.

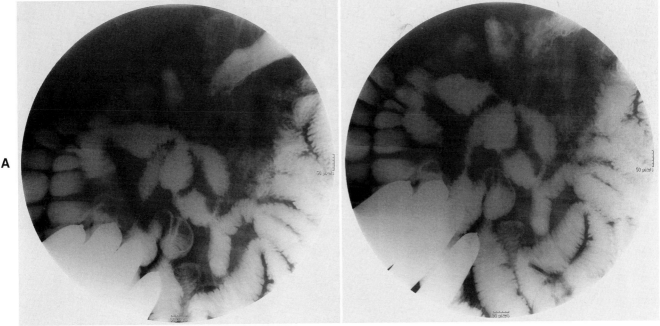

A   **B**

Courtesy Eric Bowlus, RT(R), Phoenix.

1. What causes pipelike narrowing in the small bowel?

2. The images demonstrate the pipelike narrowing referred to as what "sign"?

Chapter **5** **Gastrointestinal System**

3. When the lesions are seen with normal small bowel separation, they are referred to as

_____.

4. The combination of these signs is referred to as which disorder?

5. The radiologist has a lead glove on and is pressing on the abdomen. Why?

6. If the lesions progress, the hallmark of this disease will occur. This would be:

CASE STUDY 3

A 7-month-old male patient entered the emergency room. The history involves continued crying for the last 12 hours. A routine barium enema was performed and is presented below.

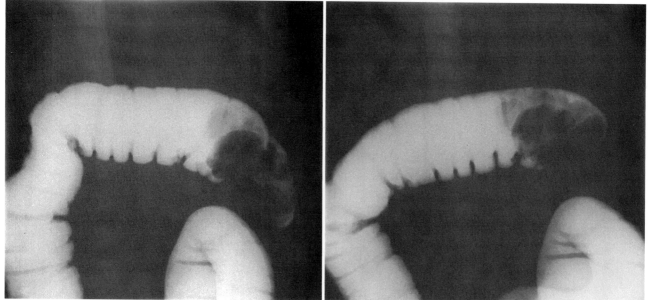

A   B

Courtesy Eric Bowlus, RT(R), Phoenix.

1. On image A, the bowel has a "coiled-spring" sign. What is this suggestive of?

2. Describe this disease process and why the "coiled-spring" sign appears.

3. What has started to occur on image B?

4. When performing a barium enema, where should the enema bag be?

   Why is this especially important?

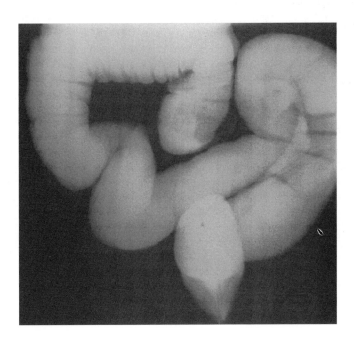

Courtesy Eric Bowlus, RT(R), Phoenix.

Chapter **5** **Gastrointestinal System**

5. This image on the preceding page demonstrates that what has occurred?

6. In this case, would the barium enema be considered diagnostic and/or therapeutic?

CASE STUDY 4

A 6-year-old patient entered the emergency room with chest and abdominal pain. A routine chest series was performed. The following is the posteroanterior upright chest image for evaluation.

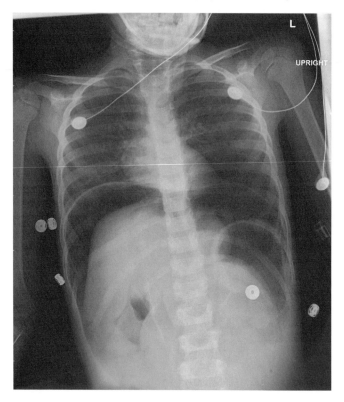

Courtesy Nicole Hightower, RT(R), Phoenix.

1. What structures demonstrate upright positioning was done besides the labeling?

Chapter 5 Gastrointestinal System

2. How long does the patient have to be in the upright position for air-fluid levels to become evident?

3. To assure that adequate time passes before completing the upright image, what is the first step the technologist should perform in this procedure?

4. If the patient arrives in the department in a wheelchair for recumbent and upright images of the chest and abdomen, which image(s) should be completed first? Why?

5. Is any free air demonstrated on this image? If so, where is it located?

6. What condition does this patient have?

7. If an upright position is not possible, the technologist should perform what alternate projection?

SELF-TEST

Read each question carefully, then circle the best answer.
1. Regional enteritis is also called
    a. Barrett's disease
    b. Cushing disease
    c. Crohn's disease
    d. Zollinger-Ellison disease

2. What disease is known for demonstrating the pathologic disorder known as the "string sign"?
    a. Crohn's disease
    b. esophageal varices
    c. paralytic ileus
    d. ulcerative colitis

3. The term for outpouchings along the walls of the bowel lumen is
   a. ulcer
   b. diverticula
   c. polyp
   d. fibrosis

4. The codition of large amounts of air in dilated loops of large and small bowel is referred to as
   a. colonic ileus
   b. ischemic ileus
   c. localized ileus
   d. paralytic ileus

5. The classic appearance of annular carcinoma of the colon is a(n)
   a. apple core
   b. bird's nest
   c. eggshell
   d. ground glass

6. Varicose veins of the rectum are
   a. diverticula
   b. fibroids
   c. hemorrhoids
   d. polyps

7. The condition of the bowel telescoping into itself is
   a. herniation
   b. ileus
   c. intussusception
   d. volvulus

8. The stepladder sign is indicative of
   a. adynamic ileus
   b. paralytic ileus
   c. regional enteritis
   d. small bowel obstruction

9. The major cause of cirrhosis in the United States and Europe is
   a. alcoholism
   b. elevated cholesterol
   c. hepatitis
   d. overweight populations

10. If the patient is too ill to stand, what position should the patient be placed in to demonstrate pneumoperitoneum?
    a. right lateral decubitus, patient on their right side
    b. right lateral decubitus, patient on their left side
    c. left lateral decubitus, patient on their right side
    d. left lateral decubitus, patient on their left side

11. Twisting of the bowel upon itself is
    a. adynamic ileus
    b. volvulus
    c. intussusception
    d. regional enteritis

12. A colonic intussusception can sometimes be reduced by which radiographic procedure?
    a. CT
    b. small bowel series
    c. barium enema
    d. enteroclysis

13. The medical term denoting difficulty swallowing is
    a. deglutition
    b. dysphagia
    c. dyspnea
    d. mastication

14. An abnormal connection between the esophagus and trachea is called a(n)
    a. fistula
    b. malformation
    c. achalasia
    d. atresia

15. The "string-of-beads" appears on upright abdominal images in
    a. colonic ileus
    b. mechanical bowel obstruction
    c. paralytic bowel obstruction
    d. paralytic ileus

16. A loss of haustral markings and deep ulcerations surrounded by intraluminal gas is indicative of
    a. infectious colitis
    b. ischemic colitis
    c. regional colitis
    d. ulcerative colitis

17. Malignant polyps tend to be
    a. irregular and pedunculated
    b. irregular and sessile
    c. smooth and pedunculated
    d. smooth and sessile

18. Enzymes to aid in the digestion of proteins are produced by the
    a. duodenal bulb
    b. liver
    c. pancreas
    d. stomach

19. The milky-white product found in the stomach is
    a. chyme
    b. hydrochloric acid
    c. gastric enzymes
    d. bile

20. Any symptomatic condition or structural changes due to reflux of stomach content into the esophagus is
    a. hiatal hernia
    b. gastric ulcer
    c. GERD
    d. esophageal carcinoma

21. Inflammation of the stomach presenting as an abnormal surface pattern in the gastric mucosa is suggestive of
    a. acute gastritis
    b. chronic atrophic gastritis
    c. peptic ulcer
    d. duodenal ulcer

22. An outpouching of the posterior wall of the esophagus is considered
    a. a traction diverticulum
    b. a Zenker's diverticulum
    c. an esophageal polyp
    d. Mallory-Weiss syndrome

23. When cholesterol and pigment sediment blocks the common bile duct, causing an inflammatory attack, it is known as
    a. cholelithiasis
    b. acute cholecystitis
    c. chronic cholecystitis
    d. acute pancreatitis

24. A functional obstruction of the distal esophagus due to incomplete relaxation of the lower esophageal sphincter is
    a. achalasia
    b. Barrett's disease
    c. hiatal hernia
    d. due to ingestion of corrosive agents

25. A "donut-shaped" lesion on a transverse sonogram of the intestine is suspicious of a(n)
    a. adynamic ileus
    b. hernia
    c. intussusception
    d. volvulus

6 Urinary System

OBJECTIVES

In addition to the objectives listed at the beginning of Chapter 6 in the textbook, the user should be able to:

1. Identify anatomic structures on diagrams and radiographs of the urinary system.
2. Describe the physiology of the urinary system.
3. Differentiate the pathologic disorders of the urinary system by defining the disease processes and their radiographic manifestations.
4. Determine changes in technical factors to obtain optimal-quality radiographs for patients with various underlying pathologic conditions.

EXERCISE 1—LABELING: ANATOMY

Identify the anatomic structures indicated by writing the correct name in the space provided.
A, Location of the urinary system.

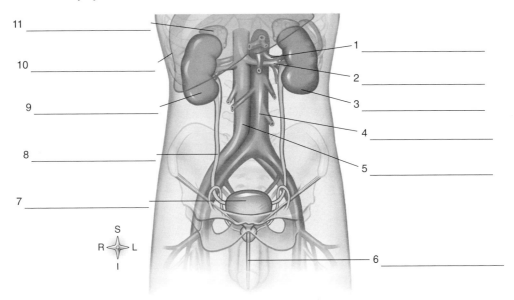

From Abrahams P, Hutchings RT, Marks SC: *McMinn's color atlas of human anatomy,* ed 4, St Louis, 1999, Mosby.

B, Internal structure of the kidney.

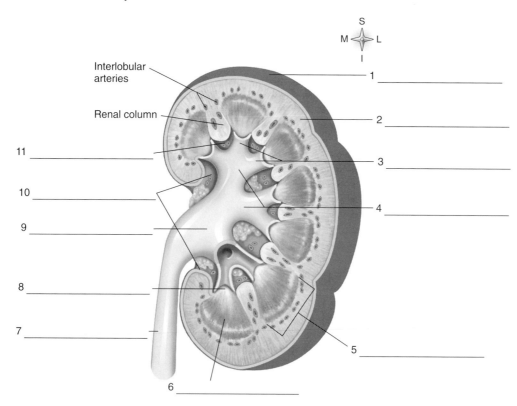

Interlobular arteries

Renal column

11 _____

10 _____

9 _____

8 _____

7 _____

6 _____

S
M ◆ L
I

1 _____

2 _____

3 _____

4 _____

5 _____

From Brundage DJ: *Renal disorders,* St Louis, 1992, Mosby.

C, Structure and location of the male urinary bladder.

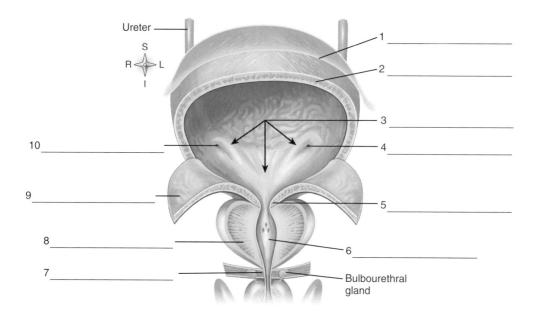

Ureter

S
R ◆ L
I

10 _____

9 _____

8 _____

7 _____

1 _____

2 _____

3 _____

4 _____

5 _____

6 _____

Bulbourethral gland

From Thibodeau GA, Patton KT: *Anatomy and physiology,* ed 6, St Louis, 2007, Mosby Elsevier.

EXERCISE 2—FILL IN THE BLANK: ANATOMY AND PHYSIOLOGY

Complete the following questions by writing the correct term(s) in the blank(s) provided.

1. The main function of the kidney is to filter the _____ from the blood and _____ water and nutrients, and _____ excess substances.

2. The functional unit of the kidney is the _____.

3. The formation of urine begins in the _____.

4. The _____ _____ _____ is where virtually all nutrients are reabsorbed into the blood capillaries.

5. The loop of Henle is a complex structure consisting of what three structures?

   a. _____

   b. _____

   c. _____

6. The kidney helps to maintain _____ balance and _____ balance of blood and body fluids.

7. The urine passes from the collecting tubules, which open into the _____.

8. From the calyces, the urine passes into the _____ _____.

9. The bladder acts as a _____ for urine until it leaves the body.

10. On the posterior aspect of the bladder, there are three openings where the _____, _____, and _____ enter or exit.

11. The triangle-shaped area on the floor of the bladder is called the _____.

12. The bladder when full is stimulated by the autonomic nervous system to produce a sensation to _____ or _____.

13. When the bladder contracts, the urine travels through the _____, exiting the body.

14. The _____ _____ prevents urine from flowing retrograde into the ureter.

15. Involuntary emptying of the bladder is referred to as _____.

EXERCISE 3—FILL IN THE BLANK: URINARY PATHOLOGY

Complete the following questions by writing the correct term(s) in the blank(s) provided.

1. When one kidney must perform the function normally carried out by two kidneys, it is a phenomenon called _____ _____.

2. The kidney position in relationship to the psoas muscle on radiographs presents as elongated or foreshortened in cases in which the kidney has _____.

Chapter **6** **Urinary System**

3. A contrast-filled _____ appears as a round or oval density surrounded by a thin radiolucent halo representing the wall of the prolapsed ureter.

4. The term for more than one ureter or renal pelvis is _____.

5. Ultrasound demonstrates the lower poles of the kidney fused, resulting in a _____

_____.

6. In chronic _____, the kidneys are bilaterally smaller with normal contours.

7. The spread of _____ to the renal pyramid causes an ulcerative, destructive process with irregularity and enlargement of the calyces.

8. The necrotic process in _____ _____ causes cavitations in the central portion of the papillae.

9. Noncontrast helical computed tomography (CT) is the safest method to demonstrate _____

_____.

10. The renal calculus that fills the renal calyces and pelvis is called a _____ calculus.

11. When a blockage in the ureter occurs above the bladder, it may cause a _____.

12. Name the four normal points of narrowing that are common sites of obstruction in the urinary system.

    a. _____

    b. _____

    c. _____

    d. _____

13. The most common unifocal mass of the kidney is a _____.

14. A multilobulated contour due to multiple cysts in the parenchyma is _____

_____ disease.

15. The triad of symptoms in renal carcinoma includes

    a. _____

    b. _____

    c. _____

16. Renal enlargement or localized bulging with elongation of adjacent calyces in an excretory urogram is suggestive

    of _____ _____.

17. Displacement and distortion of the pelvicalyceal system occur in _____

_____.

18. A plain radiograph showing punctate, coarse, or linear calcifications, usually on the periphery of the bladder, is

    suggestive of _____.

76

19. Lack of visualization of the renal vein on CT is indicative of _____

_____ _____.

20. Underlying causes of _____ _____ include bilateral renal stenosis, bilateral ureteral obstruction, and intrinsic renal disorders.

EXERCISE 4—MATCHING: ANATOMY AND PHYSIOLOGY

Match each of the following terms with the correct definition by placing the letter of the best answer in the space provided. Each question has only one correct answer. Please note that there are more terms than definitions.

1. _____ area of kidney that the blood vessels, renal pelvis, and nerves enter and exit the kidney

2. _____ carries the urine from the kidney to the bladder

3. _____ complex structure consisting of a descending limb, loop, and ascending limb

4. _____ cup-shaped top of a nephron that surrounds the glomerulus

5. _____ muscular structure on the posterior aspect of the bladder

6. _____ process of voiding

7. _____ provides the path for urine to exit the body

8. _____ stores urine before entrance into the renal pelvis

9. _____ the loop of Henle keeps a balance of salts in the body

10. _____ tuft of capillaries with very thin walls and a large surface area

11. _____ uncontrolled response of voiding

12. _____ urine passes into the papillae through this structure

A. acid-base balance

B. Bowman's capsule

C. collecting tubules

D. electrolyte balance

E. glomerulus

F. hilum

G. incontinence

H. loop of Henle

I. major calyces

J. micturition

K. proximal convoluted tubule

L. renal pelvis

M. trigone

N. ureter

O. urethra

Match each of the following terms with the correct definition by placing the letter of the best answer in the space provided. Each question has only one correct answer. Please note that there are more terms than definitions.

1. _____ eighty percent contains enough calcium to be radiopaque

2. _____ a third kidney

3. _____ cystic dilatation of the distal ureter

4. _____ destructive process involving the medullary papillae and the terminal renal pyramids

5. _____ dilatation of the renal pelvicalyceal area

6. _____ dilatation of the ureter

7. _____ ectopic kidney found in the pelvis

8. _____ evidence of a solitary kidney

9. _____ extension of a clot from the inferior vena cava

10. _____ fingerlike projections into the lumen of the bladder

11. _____ fluid-filled unilocular mass

12. _____ inflammation of the urinary bladder

13. _____ inflammatory process involving the tufts of the capillaries that filter the blood

14. _____ lesion arising from embryonic renal tissue most commonly found in infants and during childhood

15. _____ lower poles of the left and right kidneys are fused

16. _____ most common renal neoplasm, also known as a hypernephroma

17. _____ multiple cysts of varying size causing progressive renal impairment

18. _____ pyogenic bacteria causing inflammation of the kidney and renal pelvis

19. _____ results in a condition called uremia, an accumulation of excessive blood levels of urea and creatinine

20. _____ thin transverse membrane in the urethra preventing micturition

A. acute renal failure

B. bladder carcinoma

C. chronic renal failure

D. cystitis

E. glomerulonephritis

F. horseshoe kidney

G. hydronephrosis

H. hydroureter

I. papillary necrosis

J. polycystic kidney

K. positioning anomaly

L. posterior urethral valves

M. pyelonephritis

N. renal agenesis

O. renal carcinoma

P. renal cyst

Q. renal vein thrombus

R. supernumerary kidney

S. ureterocele

T. urinary calculi

U. Wilms' tumor

Circle the best answer for the following multiple choice questions.

1. A miniature replica of a normal kidney with good function is a
   a. compensatory kidney
   b. hypoplastic kidney
   c. supernumerary kidney
   d. hyperplastic kidney

2. A kidney that is not located in the retroperitoneal space adjacent to the psoas muscle is considered
   a. an ectopic kidney
   b. a compensatory kidney
   c. a hypertrophic kidney
   d. a horseshoe kidney

3. The modality to demonstrate the fused inferior poles of the kidneys without radiation exposure is
   a. CT
   b. ultrasound (US)
   c. magnetic resonance imaging (MRI)
   d. intravenous urography (IVU)

4. The _____ is a thin membrane that prevents normal urine flow.
   a. posterior urethral valve
   b. ureteropelvic junction
   c. ureterovesical junction
   d. ureterocele

5. A horseshoe kidney
   a. is lower-pole parenchymal fusion
   b. indicates a supernumerary kidney
   c. is a duplication of the ureters and renal pelvis
   d. indicates an out of position kidney

6. A dilatation of the ureter at the ureterovesical junction is a
   a. ureterocele
   b. urethral valve
   c. posterior urethral valve
   d. duplicated renal pelvis

7. Chronic pyelonephritis causes the kidneys to
   a. diminish in size
   b. have irregular contours and clubbing of the calyces
   c. produce radiolucent gas shadows within and around the kidney
   d. necrose in the central portion of the papillae

8. Small granulomas scattered in the cortices of the kidney occurs in the hematogenous spread of
   a. glomerulonephritis
   b. nephritis
   c. polynephritis
   d. tuberculosis

9. Gas-forming bacteria on plain images appearing as a lucent ring outlining all or part of the bladder are suggestive of
   a. emphysematous cystitis
   b. emphysematous pyelonephritis
   c. tuberculosis
   d. urinary calculi

10. The composition of urinary calculi can be
    a. calcium
    b. oxalates
    c. sodium
    d. a or b

11. The minuscule deposits of calcium within the renal parenchyma are
    a. urinary calculi
    b. renal calculi
    c. nephrocalcinosis
    d. tuberculosis

12. Hydronephrosis is commonly caused by
    a. a kidney stone
    b. sodium carbonate
    c. lack of peristalsis
    d. an overload of potassium

13. The modality or procedure of choice to differentiate fluid-filled simple cysts from a solid mass is
    a. CT
    b. Excretory urography
    c. kidney-ureter-bladder (KUB)
    d. US

14. The "Swiss cheese" pattern in the kidney is caused by
    a. a renal cyst
    b. innumerable lucent cysts
    c. multiple tumors
    d. nephrocalcinosis

79

15. A renal carcinoma demonstrates as a solid mass with numerous internal echoes and no evidence of acoustic enhancement when imaged with
    a. CT
    b. Excretory urography
    c. MRI
    d. US

16. In acute renal failure, the US will demonstrate
    a. atrophic kidneys
    b. intrarenal or perirenal infection
    c. postobstructive hydronephrosis
    d. renal function

17. Polypoid defects and bladder wall thickening are indicative of
    a. hypernephroma
    b. nephroblastoma
    c. bladder carcinoma
    d. cystitis

18. A highly malignant renal tumor most common in infancy and childhood is a
    a. hypernephroma
    b. renal carcinoma
    c. Wilms' tumor
    d. polycystic disease

EXERCISE 7—CASE STUDIES

The following case studies required imaging of the urinary system. After each scenario, the images are presented and you will be asked to answer questions. Using the knowledge of imaging pathology, apply exposure factors and positioning criteria to answer the questions posed.

CASE STUDY 1

A stab victim arrives in the emergency room (ER) with a puncture wound on the left posterior abdomen. A contrast-enhanced CT was completed as part of the ER work-up.

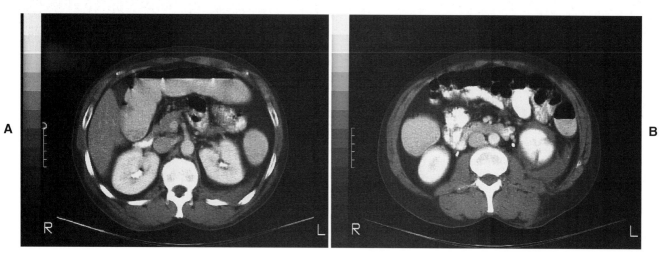

1. On CT images, the normal kidney appears with smooth contours lying lateral and anterior to the psoas muscle (image A). What differences are apparent on image B?

2. Does the contrast enhancement help delineate and differentiate the hematoma from the renal tissue? How?

3. Differential diagnosis?

Part 2 of this case is a patient who experienced blunt force trauma to the back. The CT examination was completed at 5-mm increments with contrast enhancement.

A

B

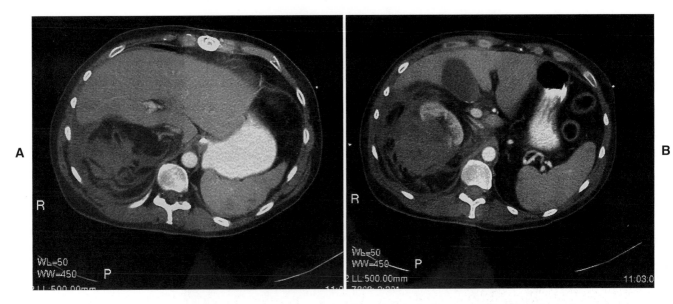

4. In image A, there appears to be pressure moving the liver anteriorly from a mass effect located posterior to the liver. Given the patient history, what does the mass possibly represent?

5. On image B, the region of the mass is associated with which anatomic structure?

6. Differential diagnosis?

A patient enters the radiography department with an order for an excretory urogram. The patient is experiencing left flank pain and has hematuria. An IVU was done, with the initial images presented below.

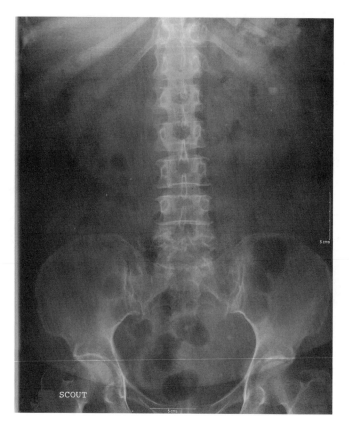

Courtesy Eric Bowlus, RT(R), Phoenix.

1. The protocol for excretory urography requires a "scout" image before beginning the contrast portion of the exam. Of what importance is the above image?

2. Is any pathology demonstrated on the scout image?

3. Once the contrast is injected, how will the pathology demonstrate?

Chapter **6 Urinary System**

Part 2 of this scenario: In another case this scout film was also the initial film for an excretory urogram and has been cropped to include only the pelvis.

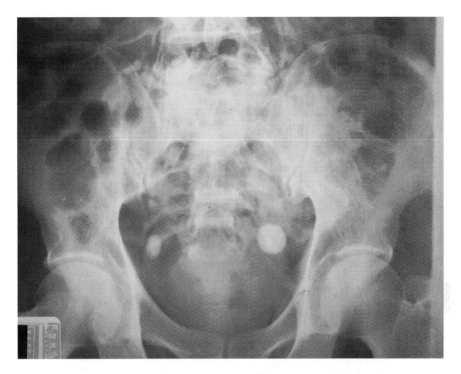

Courtesy Eric Bowlus, RT(R), Phoenix.

4. In this case, what pathology is demonstrated?

5. When contrast from the IVU enters the bladder, will the pathology be evident?

6. Differential diagnosis?

An 83-year-old male patient entered the radiology department scheduled for a cystogram. The clinical findings are to rule out bladder tracking through the inguinal canal; therefore a cystogram was the procedure of choice. A routine cystogram was performed and some images are presented below.

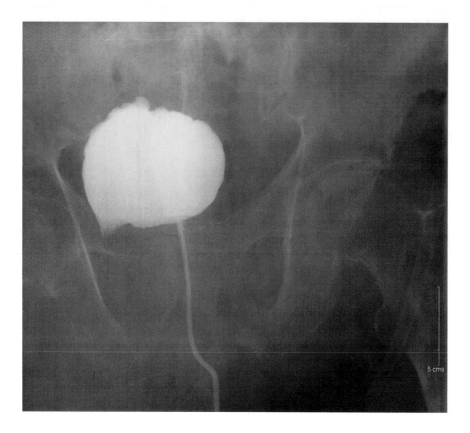

1. The tube entering the bladder represents the _____.

2. What does Image A demonstrate?

3. Does the image demonstrate any possible pathology?

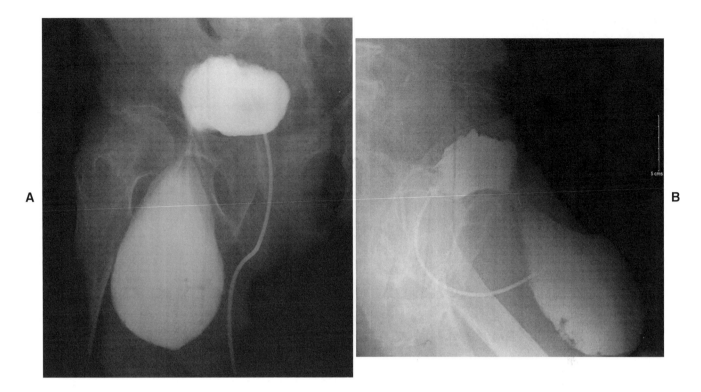

A   B

4. On the oblique image A, the contrast is located where?

5. A lateral image was taken (image B) to provide what additional information?

6. What pathologic conditions can describe these images?

SELF-TEST

Read each question carefully, then circle the best answer.
1. To assure that the diagnosis is renal agenesis, the best modality or image to demonstrate the abdomen is
   a. KUB
   b. IVU
   c. CT
   d. US

Chapter **6** **Urinary System**

2. An abnormal position of the kidney in relationship to the psoas muscle in the retroperitoneal location is considered
   a. ectopic
   b. to have malrotation
   c. hypertrophic
   d. hypoplastic

3. When IVU demonstrates two ureters exiting from one kidney, the term _____ is used.
   a. duplication
   b. fused
   c. ectopic
   d. malrotation

4. A second kidney found in the pelvis or thoracic cavity is considered a(n)
   a. ectopic kidney
   b. duplicated kidney
   c. rotated kidney
   d. fused kidney

5. A transverse membrane in the urethra demonstrates as a stricture or narrowing in a(n)
   a. ureterocele
   b. supernumerary kidney
   c. posterior urethral valve
   d. duplicated renal pelvis

6. On an excretory urogram, a characteristic ring of contrast material surrounds a triangular lucent filling defect representing the sloughed tissue in
   a. tuberculosis
   b. papillary necrosis
   c. glomerulonephritis
   d. pyelonephritis

7. Irregularity of the bladder wall and a diminished size are indicative of
   a. nephritis
   b. cystitis
   c. bladder carcinoma
   d. tuberculosis

8. Hydroureter and hydronephrosis are complications of
   a. infection in the renal cortices
   b. nephrocalcinosis
   c. obstruction due to a ureteral calculus
   d. papillary necrosis

9. Hydronephrosis can be caused by
   a. polycystic kidney disease
   b. reflux
   c. obstruction
   d. all of the above

10. Which modality or procedure best detects mass effects, stones, and other causes of obstruction?
    a. helical CT
    b. excretory urography
    c. cystogram
    d. US

11. Sonography demonstrates hydronephrosis as
    a. thickened cortices
    b. an echogenic region with acoustic shadowing
    c. echo-free sacs
    d. shadowing and swollen pyramids

12. A _____ appears as a very thin smooth radiopaque rim demonstrating the "beak sign."
    a. renal cyst
    b. renal carcinoma
    c. Wilms' tumor
    d. hypernephroma

13. To distinguish fluid-filled from solid lesions, the modality or procedure of choice is
    a. x-ray, KUB
    b. CT
    c. US
    d. x-ray, excretory urography

14. Polycystic kidney disease is(are)
    a. a fluid-filled cyst
    b. multiple cysts of varying sizes
    c. an embryonic renal mass
    d. a cyst with calcification

15. The most accurate imaging modality or procedure for detecting local and regional spread of a hypernephroma is
    a. CT
    b. US
    c. x-ray, excretory urography
    d. x-ray, KUB

16. The cobra sign is seen on an excretory urogram in the pathologic condition of
    a. posterior urethral valve
    b. renal carcinoma
    c. renal cyst
    d. ureteroceles

17. Rapid deterioration in kidney function resulting in an accumulation of waste in the blood is suggestive of
    a. acute renal failure
    b. chronic renal failure
    c. nephrocalcinosis
    d. urinary calculus

18. _____ has a triad of symptoms: hematuria, flank pain, and possibly a palpable mass.
    a. Wilms' tumor
    b. Renal carcinoma
    c. Hyperplasia
    d. Hyponephroma

19. Underlying causes for _____ include bilateral renal stenosis, bilateral ureteral obstruction, and intrinsic renal disorders.
    a. chronic renal failure
    b. renal carcinoma
    c. papillary necrosis
    d. glomerulonephritis

20. The loop of Henle keeps a balance of the salts in the body; this is a(n) _____ balance.
    a. acid-base
    b. electrolyte
    c. potassium
    d. sodium chloride

7 | Cardiovascular System

OBJECTIVES

In addition to the objectives listed at the beginning of Chapter 7 in the textbook, the user should be able to:
1. Identify anatomic structures on diagrams and radiographs of the cardiovascular system.
2. Describe the physiology of the cardiovascular system.
3. Differentiate the pathologic disorders of the cardiovascular system by defining the disease processes and their radiographic manifestations.
4. Determine changes in technical factors to obtain optimal-quality radiographs for patients with various underlying pathologic conditions.

EXERCISE 1—LABELING: ANATOMY

Identify the anatomic structures indicated by writing the correct name in the space provided.
A, Conduction system of the heart and vascular anatomy.

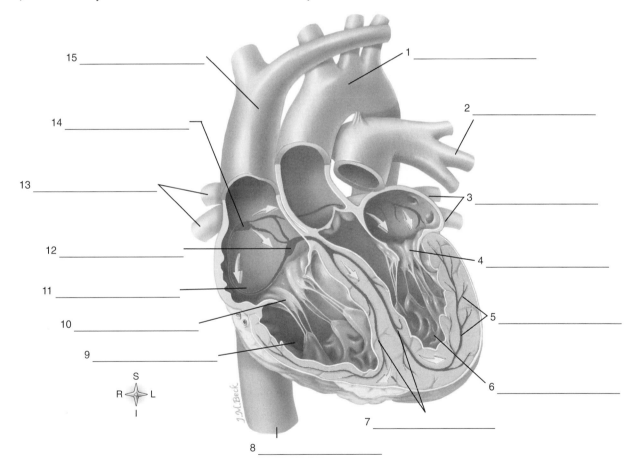

From Thibodeau GA, Patton KT: *Anatomy and physiology*, ed 6, St Louis, 2007, Mosby Elsevier.

B, Principal arteries.

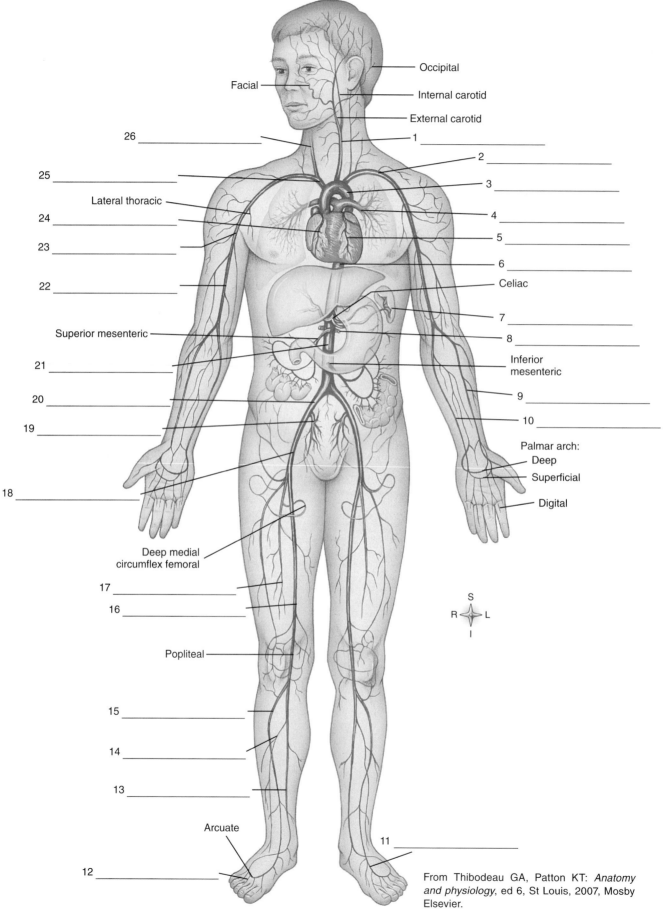

Occipital

Facial

Internal carotid

External carotid

26 _____ 1 _____

2 _____

25 _____ 3 _____

Lateral thoracic

4 _____

24 _____ 5 _____

23 _____ 6 _____

Celiac

22 _____ 7 _____

Superior mesenteric 8 _____

Inferior
mesenteric

21 _____ 9 _____

20 _____ 10 _____

19 _____

Palmar arch:
Deep
Superficial

Digital

18 _____

Deep medial
circumflex femoral

17 _____

16 _____

Popliteal

15 _____

14 _____

13 _____

Arcuate

11 _____

12 _____

From Thibodeau GA, Patton KT: *Anatomy
and physiology*, ed 6, St Louis, 2007, Mosby
Elsevier.

90

C, Structure of the heart valves.

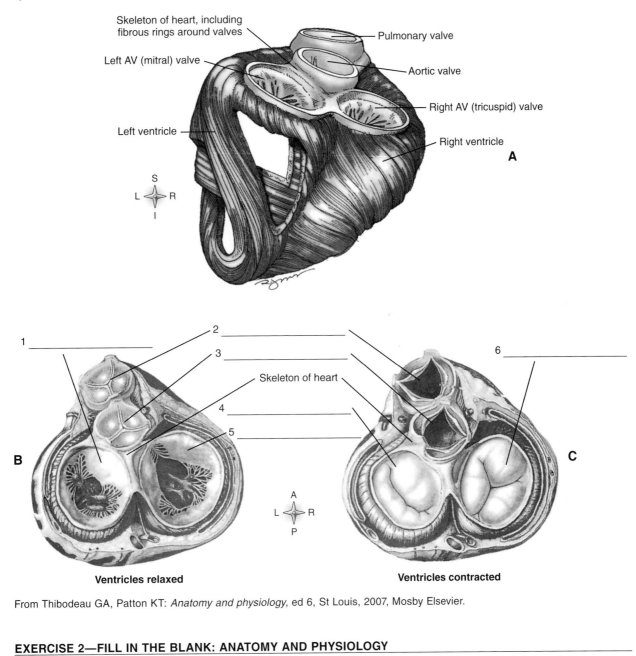

Skeleton of heart, including
fibrous rings around valves

Pulmonary valve

Left AV (mitral) valve

Aortic valve

Right AV (tricuspid) valve

Left ventricle

Right ventricle

A

S
L — R
I

1 _____

2 _____

3 _____

Skeleton of heart

4 _____

5 _____

6 _____

B

C

A
L — R
P

Ventricles relaxed

Ventricles contracted

From Thibodeau GA, Patton KT: *Anatomy and physiology*, ed 6, St Louis, 2007, Mosby Elsevier.

EXERCISE 2—FILL IN THE BLANK: ANATOMY AND PHYSIOLOGY

Complete the following questions by writing the correct term(s) in the blank(s) provided.

1. The main function of the cardiovascular system is to maintain an adequate _____ of

   _____ to all the tissues in the body.

2. The function of the cardiovascular system is accomplished by _____

   _____ of the heart.

3. The heart rate is controlled by the _____ nervous system.

4. _____ accelerates the heart rate and increases the force of its contraction.

5. Name the four chambers of the heart in order of blood entering and exiting.

   a. _____

   b. _____

   c. _____

   d. _____

6. The purpose of the heart valve is to prevent _____.

7. The heart chambers are composed of _____ _____.

8. The tricuspid valve has three _____ and is between the _____ atrium

   and the _____ ventricle.

9. The semilunar valves separate the _____ from the great vessels leaving the

   _____.

10. _____ circulation provides oxygen and nourishment to tissues throughout the body.

11. _____ circulation is the circulation of blood through the lungs to increase the oxygen level in the blood.

12. _____ circulation requires a greater pressure so the wall of the _____ ventricle is considerably thicker.

13. The heart chambers relax and fill with blood during _____.

14. The rhythm of the heart is dependent upon the conduction system, which produces impulses initially in

    the _____ _____ and _____

    _____.

EXERCISE 3—FILL IN THE BLANK: CARDIOVASCULAR PATHOLOGY

Complete the following questions by writing the correct term(s) in the blank(s) provided.

1. Diastolic overloading and enlargement of the left atrium and left ventricle are the radiographic appearance of

   _____ _____ _____.

2. _____ _____ _____ produces a prominent aortic knob because of the shunting of blood through the aorta.

3. Tetralogy of Fallot consists of a combination of what four abnormalities?

   a. _____

   b. _____

   c. _____

   d. _____

4. _____ of the aorta causes a decreased blood flow to the abdomen and legs because of the constriction of the vessel.

5. In most patients, coronary artery narrowing is caused by deposits of _____ material on the inner arterial wall.

6. Death of the myocardium due to coronary artery occlusion is referred to as a _____

_____.

7. Fifty percent of coronary artery disease occurs in the _____ coronary.

8. In percutaneous transluminal coronary angioplasty, a balloon catheter is used to _____ the constricted coronary artery.

9. Name the four associated radiographic appearances related to left-sided heart failure.

a. _____

b. _____

c. _____

d. _____

10. The radiographer can influence the size of the heart on an image by changing which three positioning criteria?

a. _____

b. _____

c. _____

11. Cardiomegaly is evaluated using the _____ ratio.

12. The most common cause of pulmonary edema is elevated _____

_____ pressure.

13. A loss of normal sharp definition of the pulmonary vascular markings occurs in _____

_____.

14. Blood pressure is dependent upon what two factors?

a. _____

b. _____

15. Name the two types of aneurysms.

a. _____

b. _____

16. A kidney-ureter-bladder (KUB) demonstrates a curvilinear _____ in the wall of an aneurysm.

17. Abdominal aortic aneurysms are called the "silent killer" because of the danger of a _____

_____.

18. In cases of closed chest trauma, name the other imaging signs besides mediastinal widening that are important for a definitive diagnosis of rupture of the aorta.

    a. _____

    b. _____

    c. _____

19. An intravascular clot is called a(n) _____.

20. _____ is the most sensitive and most specific noninvasive method for diagnosing mitral stenosis.

EXERCISE 4—MATCHING: ANATOMY AND PHYSIOLOGY

Match each of the following terms with the correct definition by placing the letter of the best answer in the space provided. Each question has only one correct answer. Please note that there are more terms than definitions.

1. _____ chambers receiving blood from the great vessels

2. _____ circulation providing the myocardium with nourishment

3. _____ circulatory process of oxygenating the blood and removing waste products

4. _____ contraction phase of the heart

5. _____ double membranous sac surrounding the heart

6. _____ excitable components with the ability to create impulses

7. _____ four chambers composed of myocardium

8. _____ larger and thicker chambers providing circulation of the blood

9. _____ prevents back flow between the right atrium and right ventricle

10. _____ provides the body with blood

11. _____ separates the ventricles and the great vessels leaving the heart

12. _____ stimulate mechanical contraction of the atria

A. atria

B. atrioventricular (AV) node

C. conduction system

D. coronary circulation

E. diastole

F. heart

G. intrinsic rhythm

H. mitral valve

I. pericardium

J. pulmonary circulation

K. semilunar valve

L. sinoatrial (SA) node

M. systemic circulation

N. systole

O. tricuspid valve

P. ventricles

Match each of the following terms with the correct definition by placing the letter of the best answer in the space provided. Each question has only one correct answer. Please note that there are more terms than definitions.

1. _____ abnormal accumulation of fluid in the extravascular tissue

2. _____ accumulation of fluid within the space surrounding the heart

3. _____ closed chest trauma with mediastinal widening

4. _____ develop in the veins where blood flow is static (or slow)

5. _____ diffuse thickening of the valve by fibrous tissue or calcific deposits

6. _____ dilated elongated tortuous vessels

7. _____ disruption of the inner layer of the blood vessel allowing blood to enter the wall of the aorta

8. _____ fatty material of the inner arterial wall

9. _____ free communication between the atria from the lack of closure of the foramen ovale

10. _____ generalized tortuosity and elongation of the ascending aorta

11. _____ inability of the heart to provide the body with an adequate blood supply

12. _____ leading cause of strokes and congestive heart failure

13. _____ most common cause of cyanotic congenital heart disease

14. _____ narrowing or arteries causes oxygen deprivation of the myocardium

15. _____ narrowing or constriction of the aorta

16. _____ obstruction of the left ventricular outflow increases the workload of the left ventricle

17. _____ part or all of the clot becomes detached from the vessel wall

18. _____ saccular and fusiform are types

19. _____ symptom of hardened arteries that have a loss of elasticity

20. _____ vessel connecting the pulmonary artery and the aorta

A. aneurysm

B. aortic dissection

C. aortic rupture

D. aortic stenosis

E. atherosclerosis

F. atrial septal defect

G. coarctation of the aorta

H. congestive heart failure

I. coronary artery disease

J. embolism

K. hypertension

L. hypertensive heart disease

M. infective endocarditis

N. mitral insufficiency

O. mitral stenosis

P. patent ductus arteriosus

Q. pericardial effusion

R. plaque

S. pulmonary edema

T. rheumatic heart disease

U. tetralogy of Fallot

V. thrombosis

W. varicose veins

X. ventricular septal defect

Circle the best answer for the following multiple choice questions.

1. The most common congenital cardiac lesion is
   a. atrial septal defect
   b. patent ductus arteriosus
   c. ventricular septal defect
   d. tetralogy of Fallot

2. _____ is becoming the modality of choice to image congenital heart disease because both the morphologic and functional anomalies can be visualized.
   a. computed tomography (CT)
   b. ultrasound (US)
   c. magnetic resonance imaging (MRI)
   d. nuclear medicine (NM)

3. The classic "coeur en sabot" resembling the curved-toe portion of the wooden shoe appears in cases of
   a. tetralogy of Fallot
   b. coarctation
   c. patent ductus arteriosus
   d. atrial septal defect

4. Coarctation of the aorta demonstrates radiographically as
   a. rib notching and two bulges in the region of the aortic knob
   b. an enlarged heart
   c. an enlarged left atrium and ventricle
   d. "coeur en sabot"

5. The most commonly used noninvasive study to assess regional blood flow and tissue viability of the myocardium is
   a. CT
   b. MRI
   c. NM perfusion scan
   d. coronary arteriography

6. The definitive procedure to determine the presence and severity of coronary artery disease is
   a. CT
   b. computed radiography
   c. NM perfusion scan
   d. coronary arteriography

7. Right-sided heart failure causes
   a. a lack of blood flow to the organs
   b. a lack of blood flow into the systemic circulation
   c. a lack of blood flow to the extremities
   d. a back flow of blood in the venous systemic circulation

8. The "butterfly" or "bat's wings" pattern that is most prominent in the central portion of the lungs is indicative of
   a. pulmonary effusion
   b. pulmonary edema
   c. congestive heart failure
   d. aortic coarctation

9. Of the following blood pressures, which represents hypertension?
   a. 120/90
   b. 130/80
   c. 140/70
   d. 150/100

10. The "string-of-beads" pattern on a renal arteriogram suggests
    a. fibromuscular dysplasia
    b. emphysematous pyelonephritis
    c. atherosclerosis
    d. coarctation

11. A result of long-standing hypertension is
    a. atherosclerosis
    b. fibromuscular dysplasia
    c. hypertensive heart disease
    d. dilated arteries

12. Localized dilatation of an artery is a(n)
    a. aneurysm
    b. dissection
    c. rupture
    d. embolism

13. Which of the following is(are) types of aneurysms?
    a. saccular
    b. fusiform
    c. weakness in the blood vessel wall
    d. all of the above

14. For abdominal aortic aneurysms, the noninvasive modality or procedure of choice for initial detection is
    a. arteriography
    b. CT
    c. MRI
    d. US

15. To best demonstrate the location and extent of an aneurysm, the diagnostician's choice in imaging is
    a. CTA
    b. MRA
    c. US
    d. Either a or b

16. _____ begins with an intimal tear in the aorta.
    a. Dissection
    b. Traumatic rupture
    c. Aneurysm
    d. Atherosclerosis

17. The classic "double-barrel" aorta is indicative of
    a. aortic rupture
    b. hypertension
    c. aortic dissection
    d. atherosclerosis

18. Fatty deposits in the artery cause
    a. plaques
    b. hemorrhages
    c. ruptures
    d. tears

19. To demonstrate venous patency in varicose veins, _____ is the procedure of choice.
    a. CTA of the lower legs
    b. lower leg venography
    c. MRA of the lower extremities
    d. lower leg angiography

20. Bacteria or fungi form vegetations on the heart valves in
    a. infective carditis
    b. rheumatic heart disease
    c. mitral stenosis
    d. mitral insufficiency

EXERCISE 7—CASE STUDIES

The following case studies required imaging related to the cardiovascular system. After each scenario, the images are presented and you will be asked to answer questions. Using the knowledge of imaging pathology, apply exposure factors and positioning criteria to answer the questions posed.

An adult male patient in the cardiac intensive care unit is experiencing SOB (shortness of breath).
A portable chest x-ray is ordered.

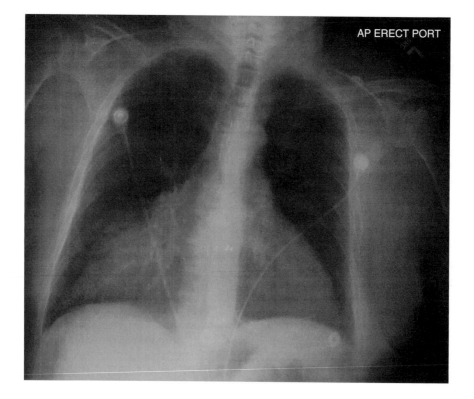

1. How was the patient positioned for this image?

    What evidence is provided to know the patient position?

2. How does the positioning in this case influence heart size?

    Will the radiologist realize that the change in the position has occurred? How?

3. What other positioning factors could cause changes in the heart size?

4. What disease process may be misdiagnosed if the radiographer does not label the image properly?

5. How large should the heart appear on an image?

Does the heart appear to be of normal size and shape? Describe the changes, if any.

6. What ratio is used to determine if the heart is enlarged?

In this case, the patient has had a heart transplant. The image provided without a history, comparison images, or proper labeling could be misdiagnosed. The image was compared with a previous image for the most accurate diagnosis. In this case, the image is considered normal for this patient. The shadow on the right, which looks like an enlarged heart, is the patient's original heart.

A patient enters the CT department with an order for an abdominal scan to rule out abdominal aortic aneurysm.

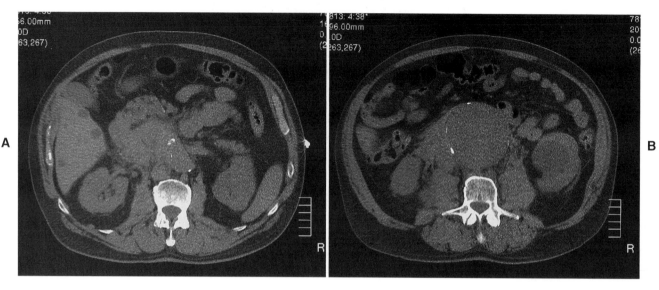

Courtesy Richard Fucillo, RT(R), Corvallis, Ore.

1. The aorta is anatomically located anterior to the spine and normally appears as an oval area slightly to the left. In this instance, is the aorta seen as described?

2. There is a mass located anterior to the spine that has small white spots embedded. What represents white on CT images and might be found in the walls of a blood vessel (the aorta)?

3. Could these deposits be seen on an abdominal image?

4. In image B, the diameter of the aorta demonstrates _____, with a hematoma (on the left and posterior, seen with soft tissue attenuation but has a very ragged edge).

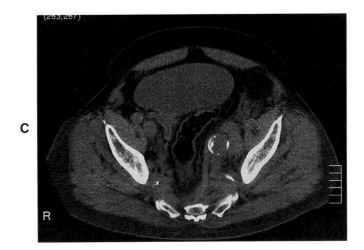

C

R

Courtesy Richard Fucillo, RT(R), Corvallis, Ore.

5. The anatomic structures represent what region of the abdomen on image C?

6. What are the arteries in this area (image C)?

7. Do the same deposits appear? Where?

CT has the ability to identify the location and extent of an abdominal aortic aneurysm. The width of the abdominal aortic aneurysm in this case is 9 cm. Contrast was not required, which is an advantage over traditional angiography.

SELF-TEST

Read each question carefully, then circle the best answer.
  1. Varicose veins usually involve the
     a. deep veins
     b. external arteries
     c. internal arteries
     d. superficial veins

2. DVT (deep vein thrombosis) can be caused by
   a. electrolyte imbalance
   b. oral contraceptives
   c. exercise
   d. diet

3. For diagnosing DVT, using an noninvasive approach, the modality with a 95% accuracy is
   a. CTA
   b. MRA
   c. duplex color Doppler US
   d. venography

4. On echocardiography, a posterior sonolucent fluid collection surrounding the heart is suggestive of
   a. pericardial effusion
   b. pleural edema
   c. pleural effusion
   d. pulmonary edema

5. The development of nodules or vegetations on the heart valves caused by bacteria or fungi is indicative of
   a. rheumatic fever
   b. pericarditis
   c. mitral stenosis
   d. infective carditis

6. _____ is a disorder that can be caused by syphilis, infective carditis, a dissection aneurysm, or Marfan syndrome.
   a. Aortic insufficiency
   b. Mitral insufficiency
   c. Mitral stenosis
   d. Rheumatic fever

7. Regurgitation indicates a(n)
   a. back flow of blood
   b. dilation of a blood vessel
   c. stenosis of a vessel
   d. infection has inflamed a vessel

8. Valve insufficiency occurs in patients with
   a. pericardial effusion
   b. rheumatic heart disease
   c. aneurysms
   d. poor cardiac output

9. A complication of infective carditis is
   a. mitral insufficiency
   b. pericardial effusion
   c. rheumatic heart disease
   d. septic emboli

10. The most common underlying disorder causing renovascular hypertension is
    a. fibromuscular dysplasia
    b. arteriosclerosis
    c. atherosclerosis
    d. aortic aneurysm

11. An aortic dissection is a
    a. hemorrhage into the mediastinum
    b. rupture of the aorta
    c. tear in the intima
    d. tear in the muscularis

12. A hemorrhage into the mediastinum causes a mediastinal widening and a loss of a discrete aortic knob shadow in a
    a. dissection of the aorta
    b. traumatic aortic rupture
    c. abdominal aortic aneurysm
    d. hypertensive heart disease

13. To identify a clot within an aneurysm, the modality of choice is
    a. abdominal aortogram
    b. CTA
    c. Doppler US
    d. none of the above

14. A saccular aneurysm is defined as a(n)
    a. inward vascular growth
    b. enlarged vessel circumference
    c. outpouching only on one side of the artery
    d. fatty deposit

15. Fatty deposits in the artery cause
    a. plaques
    b. hemorrhages
    c. ruptures
    d. tears

16. A weakness in the wall of an artery causing a dilatation is evidence of a(n)
    a. plaque
    b. aneurysm
    c. dissection
    d. rupture

17. The continued strain of _____ leads to dilatation and enlargement of the left ventricle.
    a. hypertensive heart disease
    b. fibromuscular dysplasia
    c. dissection of the aorta
    d. pulmonary emboli

18. In hypertensive heart disease, the narrowing of the systemic circulation causes
    a. an aneurysm
    b. high blood pressure
    c. the left ventricle to assume an increased workload
    d. the right ventricle's workload to increase

103

19. _____ is most commonly seen in young women and appears radiographically as a pattern of a "string of beads."
    a. Hypertension
    b. Fibrous dysplasia
    c. Hypertensive heart disease
    d. Atherosclerosis

20. Essential hypertension characterized by a gradual onset and a prolonged course is a
    a. secondary form
    b. malignant form
    c. idiopathic form
    d. benign form

21. _____ refers to an abnormal accumulation of fluid in the extravascular pulmonary tissue.
    a. Pulmonary emboli
    b. Pulmonary effusion
    c. Pulmonary edema
    d. Hypertensive heart disease

22. A bilateral symmetric fan-shaped infiltration seen on a posteroanterior chest x-ray is the characteristic radiographic sign of
    a. a butterfly, pulmonary edema
    b. a string of beads, fibrous dysplasia
    c. coeur en sabot, hypertensive heart disease
    d. the cobra, uterocele

23. The cardiothoracic (C/T) ratio is used to evaluate
    a. mediastinal shift
    b. heart size
    c. body rotation
    d. pulmonary edema

24. When the heart lacks the ability to adequately supply the body with blood, the patient has
    a. congestive heart failure
    b. pericardial effusion
    c. hypertensive heart disease
    d. increased cardiac output

25. When coronary vascularization is occluded, the area of the myocardium loses its blood supply, causing
    a. rheumatic heart disease
    b. myocardial infarction
    c. hypertensive heart disease
    d. congestive heart failure

26. A constriction of the aorta causing a reduced blood flow to the abdominal organs and the lower extremities is called _____ of the aorta.
    a. rupture
    b. dissection
    c. coarctation
    d. ductus arteriosus

27. Cyanotic congenital heart disease consists of four abnormalities to include high ventricular septal defect, overriding of the aortic orifice above the ventricular defect, right ventricular hypertrophy, and
   a. mitral stenosis
   b. pulmonary stenosis
   c. tricuspid stenosis
   d. aortic stenosis

28. A vessel extending from the pulmonary artery to the _____ occurs in a patient with patent ductus arteriosus.
   a. aorta
   b. pulmonary vein
   c. superior vena cava
   d. left atrium

29. Free communication between the atria is _____, which causes a left to right shunting effect.
   a. patent ductus arteriosus
   b. ventricular septal defect
   c. atrial septal defect
   d. tetralogy of Fallot

30. If the first impulse in the conduction system of the heart fails to fire, the _____ will generate rhythmic impulses at a slower than normal rate.
   a. ectopic pacemaker
   b. sinoatrial node
   c. atrioventricular node
   d. bundle of His

8 Nervous System

OBJECTIVES

In addition to the objectives listed at the beginning of Chapter 8 in the textbook, the user should be able to:

1. Identify anatomic structures on diagrams and radiographs of the nervous system.
2. Describe the physiology of the nervous system.
3. Differentiate the pathologic disorders of the nervous system by defining the disease processes and their radiographic manifestations.
4. Determine changes in technical factors to obtain optimal-quality radiographs for patients with various underlying pathologic conditions.

Identify the anatomic structures indicated by writing the correct name in the space provided.
A, Structure of a neuron.

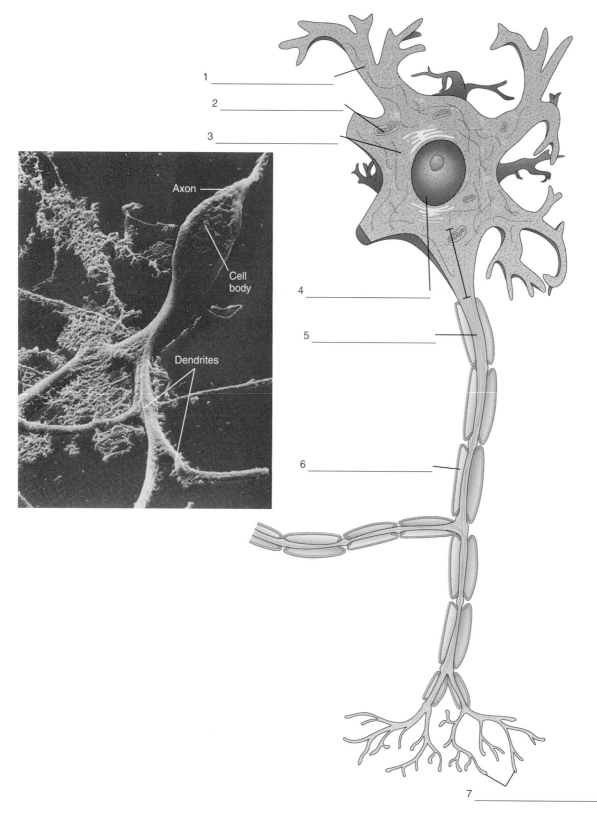

1 _____

2 _____

3 _____

4 _____

5 _____

6 _____

7 _____

Axon

Cell body

Dendrites

From Thibodeau GA, Patton KT: *Anatomy and physiology*, ed 6, St Louis, 2007, Mosby Elsevier.

B, Covering structures of the central nervous system.

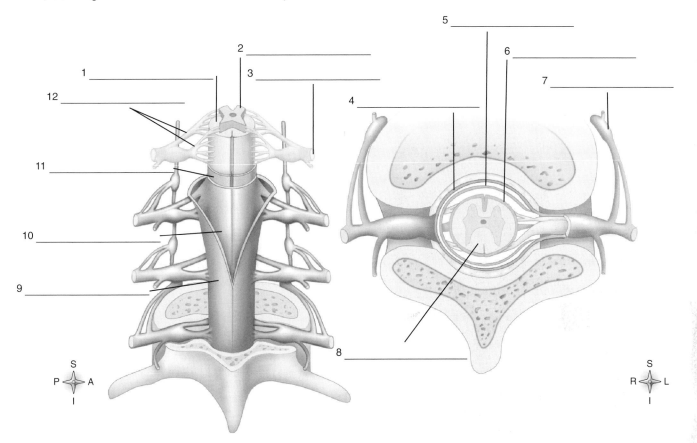

From Thibodeau GA, Patton KT: *Anatomy and physiology*, ed 6, St Louis, 2007, Mosby Elsevier.

C, Divisions of the brain.

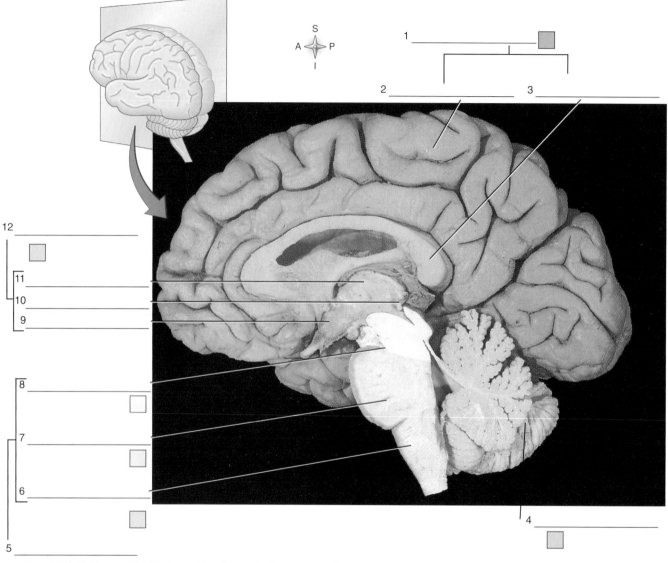

From Vidic B, Suarez FR: *Photographic atlas of the human body,* St Louis, 1984, Mosby.

EXERCISE 2—FILL IN THE BLANK: ANATOMY AND PHYSIOLOGY

Complete the following questions by writing the correct term(s) in the blank(s) provided.

1. The _____ _____ system consists of the cranial, spinal, and autonomic nerves.

2. _____ neurons, also known as sensory, carry impulses to the central nervous system from the peripheral receptors.

3. Efferent neurons conduct impulses away from the _____ to the

   _____ _____.

4. The smooth muscle, cardiac muscle, and glandular epithelial tissue are controlled by the _____ nervous system.

5. The basic unit of the nervous system is the _____.

6. A single threadlike extension, a(n) _____ leads away from the nerve cell body.

7. To increase the rate of transmission of nervous impulses, the axon is insulated by the _____ _____.

8. A chemical reaction permits the travel of impulses from the dendrite to the next axon at the _____.

9. A _____ _____ consists of the travel of an impulse from a peripheral receptor to the peripheral effectors.

10. The neurons that carry the impulse to the skeletal muscle to cause movement are called the _____ or _____ neurons.

11. The thin layer of gray matter where nerve cell bodies are concentrated is the _____ of the cerebrum.

12. The two hemispheres are called the _____.

13. High elevated convolutions on the surface of the cerebrum are the _____.

14. _____ mater is the inner area of the cerebrum consisting of nerve fiber tracts.

15. The cerebral cortex is responsible for receiving _____ information from the body and for triggering impulses to control _____ activity.

16. _____ impulses are transmitted to the posterior portion of the brain.

17. Stimulation on one side of the cerebral cortex causes contraction of muscle on the _____ side of the body.

18. The _____ _____ connects the two cerebral hemispheres by a mass of white matter.

19. The caudate nuclei, globus pallidus, and putamen make up the _____ _____.

20. The _____ is composed of the midbrain, the pons, and the medulla.

21. The coordination of muscle groups by the _____ helps to maintain equilibrium and posture.

22. The outer protective covering of the brain is the _____.

23. Name three meningeal layers, from the innermost to the outer layer.

   a. _____

   b. _____

   c. _____

24. The third and fourth ventricles are connected by the _____ of

   _____.

25. The superior portion of the third ventricle, which connects the lateral ventricles, is known as the

   _____ of _____.

26. The choroid plexus is located in the _____ ventricles and the roofs of the third and fourth
   ventricles.

27. The _____ _____ is a tentlike covering over the cerebellum that
   separates it from the occipital lobe of the cerebrum.

28. The _____ is a relay station that receives and processes sensory information.

29. Name the two divisions of the nervous system.

   a. _____

   b. _____

30. Name the three structures found in the diencephalon.

   a. _____

   b. _____

   c. _____

EXERCISE 3—FILL IN THE BLANK: NERVOUS SYSTEM PATHOLOGY

Complete the following questions by writing the correct term(s) in the blank(s) provided.

1. Mumps, polio, and possibly herpes simplex cause _____.

2. Acute inflammation of the meninges (pia mater and arachnoid) is _____.

3. Mild headaches and fever to more severe cerebral dysfunction, seizures, and a coma may result from the viral

   infection of the brain called _____.

4. The most common form of meningitis is caused by _____ _____,

   _____, and _____.

5. An area with poorly defined borders and a mass effect reflecting vascular congestion and edema represent the earli-

   est signs of a(n) _____ _____ on computed tomography (CT) and
   magnetic resonance (MR) images.

6. _____ is the procedure of choice to demonstrate a crescenteric or lentiform extraaxial fluid collection adjacent to the skull border.

7. In _____ empyema, the infectious process is localized outside the dural membrane.

8. Name the two suppurative processes of the central nervous system.

    a. _____

    b. _____

9. A _____ fracture is a linear fracture that intersects a skull suture and courses along it.

10. A stellate fracture has multiple fracture lines radiating outward from a central point, is usually found in the skull,

    and is known as a _____ fracture.

11. Name the four different types of cerebral hematomas.

    a. _____

    b. _____

    c. _____

    d. _____

12. An epidural hematoma appears as a _____ peripheral high-density lesion on a CT scan of the brain.

13. A(n) _____ hematoma demonstrates an increased density that has a crescentic shape adjacent to the inner table of the skull.

14. The frontal and anterior temporal regions are the most common site of injury demonstrating edema and hemorrhage

    in cases of _____ _____.

15. The evidence of bleeding as increased density within the basilar cisterns, cerebral fissures, and sulci indicate a(n)

    _____ _____.

16. The face consists of thin, poorly supported bones that easily _____ in response to a traumatic force.

17. The _____ fracture can be hammocklike or trap-door variety, which is best demonstrated

    on _____.

18. The submentovertex projection best demonstrates _____ _____ fractures.

19. A(n) _____ fracture results in a free-floating zygoma, causing disfiguration if not treated.

20. The angle of the _____ is the most common fracture site of the jaw.

21. The most common facial fracture is a fracture of the _____ _____.

22. Processes causing _____ _____ include abnormal vessel walls, occlusions, blood vessel ruptures, and decreased blood flow.

23. Imaging evaluation in acute strokes is to _____ or _____ other disorders that simulate the same clinical findings.

24. An embolic stroke or stenosis causing a temporary blockage of a cerebral vessel is a(n)

_____.

25. A _____ scan is used as a screening study to demonstrate the carotid artery.

26. On a fresh bleed, the CT scan demonstrates a homogeneously dense, well-defined lesion with a round to oval

configuration in cases of a(n) _____ hemorrhage.

EXERCISE 4—FILL IN THE BLANK: NERVOUS SYSTEM PATHOLOGY

Complete the following questions by writing the correct term(s) in the blank(s) provided.

1. _____ is the most sensitive technique for detecting most suspected brain tumors.

2. Seizure disorders and gradual neurologic deficits are the clinical signs of a _____ of the central nervous system.

3. A(n) _____ _____ usually originates in the internal auditory canal and extends into the cerebellopontine angle cistern.

4. A nonsecreting pituitary adenoma is called a _____ _____.

5. _____ have calcifications that usually can be detected on plain skull images.

6. Rapidly growing germ cell tumors occurring more frequently in males are the _____ and

_____.

7. Ill-defined bone destruction or cortical expansion and a flocculent calcification are the radiographic appearances

suggestive of a _____.

8. In MR, single or multiple masses presenting a high signal intensity on a T2-weighted image situated at the junction

between gray mater and white mater is _____ _____.

9. _____ _____ is the mildest type of epilepsy, which primarily occurs in children.

10. _____ is the modality of choice to localize the seizure focus in a patient with hippocampal sclerosis.

11. Ventricular dilatation with prominent sulci in the cerebral hemispheres is indicative of _____

_____.

12. Name the four characteristics of Parkinson's disease.

a. _____

b. _____

c. _____

d. _____

13. Atrophy of the caudate nucleus and putamen is the hallmark of _____ disease.

14. Name the two types of hydrocephalus.

    a. _____

    b. _____

15. Mucosal thickening most commonly seen in the maxillary antra is _____.

EXERCISE 5—MATCHING: ANATOMY

Match each of the following terms with the correct definition by placing the letter of the best answer in the space provided. Each question has only one correct answer. Please note that there are more terms than definitions.

1. _____ afferent and efferent neurons

2. _____ fatty covering providing insulation

3. _____ impulse conducted to and from

4. _____ impulses travel from the central nervous system to the peripheral effectors

5. _____ junction between neurons

6. _____ nerve cell

7. _____ one or more threadlike extensions leading toward a cell body

8. _____ supplies the striated skeletal muscles

9. _____ the brain and spinal cord

10. _____ conducts impulses from the peripheral receptors to the central nervous system

A. autonomic nervous system

B. axon

C. central nervous system

D. dendrite

E. motor neurons

F. myelin sheath

G. neuron

H. peripheral nervous system

I. reflex arc

J. sensory neurons

K. somatic nervous system

L. synapse

Match each of the following terms with the correct definition by placing the letter of the best answer in the space provided. Each question has only one correct answer. Please note that there are more terms than definitions.

1. _____ absorbs cerebrospinal fluid into the venous blood circulation

2. _____ acts with the cerebral cortex to produce skilled movements by coordinating muscle groups

3. _____ cerebrospinal fluid is housed here

4. _____ connects the two cerebral hemispheres

5. _____ controls position and automatic movement

6. _____ convoluted elevations

7. _____ deep grooves dividing cerebral hemispheres

8. _____ delicate weblike middle covering of the central nervous system

9. _____ largest part of the brain

10. _____ link between the mind and body

11. _____ outer portion of cerebrum

12. _____ produces cerebrospinal fluid

13. _____ resembles a worm coiled on itself

14. _____ separates the cerebral hemispheres

15. _____ shallow grooves

16. _____ superior portion of the brainstem

17. _____ three membranes providing protection for the central nervous system

18. _____ tough outer covering of the brain

A. aqueduct of Sylvius

B. arachnoid membrane

C. arachnoid villi

D. basal ganglia

E. cerebellum

F. cerebrum

G. choroid plexus

H. corpus callosum

I. cortex

J. diencephalon

K. dura mater

L. falx cerebelli

M. falx cerebri

N. fissures

O. foramen of Monro

P. hypothalamus

Q. gyri

R. medulla

S. meninges

T. midbrain

U. pia mater

V. pons

W. subarachnoid space

X. sulci

Y. thalamus

Z. vermis

Match each of the following terms with the correct definition by placing the letter of the best answer in the space provided. Each question has only one correct answer. Please note that there are more terms than definitions.

1. _____ acute arterial bleed commonly over the parietotemporal convexity

2. _____ almost invariably associated with osteomyelitis

3. _____ any process caused by an abnormality of the blood vessels or blood supply to the brain

4. _____ appears radiographically as multiple small poorly defined areas of lucency

5. _____ bilateral and horizontal fracture of the maxillae

6. _____ commonly caused by *Haemophilus influenzae* in neonates and young adults

7. _____ direct blow to the front of the orbit caused by a rapid increase in intraorbital pressure

8. _____ focal neurologic deficit that completely resolves in 24 hours

9. _____ fractures of the zygomatic arch, orbital floor, and a separation of the zygomaticofrontal suture

10. _____ hypertensive vascular disease causes

11. _____ injury to the surface veins, cerebral parenchyma, cortical arteries, or a rupture of an aneurysm

12. _____ loculated infection most often in the gray matter

13. _____ most commonly ruptured veins between the dura and the arachnoid

14. _____ occurs when the brain comes in contact with the rough skull surfaces

15. _____ penetrating trauma to the neck that possibly results in a traumatic fistula

16. _____ sharp lucent line

17. _____ shearing forces tearing the arteries

18. _____ sudden and dramatic development of a focal neurologic deficit

19. _____ suppurative process between the dura mater and arachnoid

20. _____ viral inflammation of the brain and meninges

A. abscess

B. bacterial meningitis

C. blowout fracture

D. carotid artery injury

E. cerebral contusion

F. cerebrovascular disease

G. encephalitis

H. epidural empyema

I. epidural hematoma

J. intracerebral hematoma

K. intraparenchymal hemorrhage

L. Le Fort fracture

M. osteomyelitis of the skull

N. sinusitis

O. skull fracture

P. stroke syndrome

Q. subarachnoid hemorrhage

R. subdural empyema

S. subdural hematoma

T. transient ischemic attack

U. tripod fracture

V. viral meningitis

Match each of the following terms with the correct definition by placing the letter of the best answer in the space provided. Each question has only one correct answer. Please note that there are more terms than definitions.

1. _____ abnormal cells reaching the brain by hematogenous spread

2. _____ arises from remnants of the embryonic neural tube most often at the clivus or lower lumbosacral region

3. _____ benign tumor having cystic and solid components originating from embryonic remnants

4. _____ causes gigantism in adolescents and acromegaly in adults

5. _____ condition of the brain in which temporary disturbances occur, causing a range of signs

6. _____ dilatation of the ventricular system

7. _____ focal or generalized enlargement of cranial nerve VIII

8. _____ generalized convulsions associated with a patient falling, hypersalivation, and incontinence (bowel and bladder)

9. _____ germinomas and teratomas are types

10. _____ involuntary movements and early dementia

11. _____ most common primary malignant brain tumor consisting of glial cells

12. _____ normal aging results in enlargement of the ventricular system and sulci, causing forgetfulness

13. _____ progressive cerebral atrophy developing at an earlier age than the senile period

14. _____ shaking palsy with stooped posture, stiffness, and slow movement with a fixed facial expression

15. _____ slow growing tumors that form large cavities or pseudocysts

16. _____ tumor arising from arachnoid lining cells and attached to the dura mater

17. _____ viral infection of upper respiratory tract

18. _____ widespread selective atrophy and loss of motor nerve cells leading to extensive paralysis

A. acoustic neuroma

B. Alzheimer's disease

C. amyotrophic lateral sclerosis

D. astrocytoma

E. cerebellar atrophy

F. chordoma

G. craniopharyngioma

H. dementia

I. epilepsy

J. glioma

K. grand mal seizures

L. Huntington's disease

M. hydrocephalus

N. meningioma

O. metastatic carcinoma

P. multiple sclerosis

Q. Parkinson's disease

R. pineal tumor

S. pituitary adenoma

T. sinusitis

Circle the best answer for the following multiple choice questions.

1. The most common form of inflammation of the pia mater and arachnoid is
   a. bacterial meningitis
   b. encephalitis
   c. viral meningitis
   d. a brain abscess

2. Which of the following is not a membrane covering the brain?
   a. dura mater
   b. pia mater
   c. arachnoid
   d. epidural

3. Brain metastases usually originate in the
   a. testicles and kidney
   b. lung and breast
   c. breast and cervix
   d. colon and lung

4. A hematoma occurring after a blunt head injury causing venous bleeding is a(n)
   a. epidural hematoma
   b. subarachnoid bleed
   c. subdural hematoma
   d. cerebral contusion

5. Movement of the brain within the calvaria following blunt trauma to the skull sometimes results in a cerebral _____.
   a. subdural hematoma
   b. epidural hematoma
   c. acute hematoma
   d. contusion

6. Which of the following is the most common cause of a brain abscess?
   a. streptococci
   b. *Haemophilus influenzae*
   c. herpes simplex
   d. sinus infection

7. Sinus radiographs should be taken using a _____ beam and with the patient in the _____ position.
   a. vertical; recumbent
   b. vertical; prone
   c. horizontal; erect
   d. vertical; erect

8. The process associated with osteomyelitis, causing a low-density poorly defined area adjacent to the inner skull table on CT, is a case of
   a. brain abscess
   b. epidural empyema
   c. subarachnoid empyema
   d. subdural empyema

9. The _____ consists of the multiplication of glial cells, which spread by direct extension.
   a. glioma
   b. meningioma
   c. acoustic neuroma
   d. pituitary adenoma

10. A(n) _____ grows slowly, arising from the Schwann cells on the eighth cranial nerve.
    a. pituitary adenoma
    b. chromophobe adenoma
    c. acoustic neuroma
    d. meningioma

11. A meningioma is a benign tumor arising from
    a. arachnoid lining cells and is attached to the dura
    b. glial cells spreading by direct extension
    c. anterior lobe of the pituitary gland
    d. embryonic remnants

12. An air-fluid level seen in the sphenoid sinus is indicative of a _____ skull fracture.
    a. basilar
    b. tripod
    c. blowout
    d. nasal bone

13. Rapidly growing germ cell tumors known as _____ are best demonstrated on MR sagittal images.
    a. pituitary tumors
    b. chordomas
    c. pineal tumors
    d. acoustic tumors

Chapter **8** **Nervous System**

14. Tumors arising from the embryonic neural tube commonly found at the clivus are considered
    a. meningiomas
    b. chordomas
    c. neuromas
    d. gliomas

15. Acute arterial bleeding most commonly caused by a laceration of the medial meningeal artery is a _____ hematoma.
    a. subarachnoid
    b. subdural
    c. epidural
    d. intracerebral

16. Le Fort fractures result in a(n)
    a. detached fragment that is unstable and altered
    b. bilateral injury at the angle
    c. zygoma detachment
    d. inferior orbital rim fracture

17. Hemorrhagic strokes are most commonly caused by
    a. a berry aneurysm
    b. hypertension
    c. carotid artery disease
    d. a and b

18. Widespread selective atrophy with loss of neuromotor function leading to paralysis is
    a. hydrocephalus
    b. Alzheimer's disease
    c. Parkinson's disease
    d. amyotrophic lateral sclerosis

19. Scattered plaques of demyelination on MR images are
    a. multiple sclerosis
    b. epilepsy
    c. Alzheimer's disease
    d. Huntington's disease

20. The essence of the condition seems to be an inadequate production of dopamine in cases of _____ disease.
    a. Huntington's
    b. Parkinson's
    c. Alzheimer's
    d. epileptic

EXERCISE 10—CASE STUDIES

The following case studies required imaging related to the nervous system. After each scenario, the images are presented and you will be asked to answer questions. Using the knowledge of imaging pathology, apply exposure factors and positioning criteria to answer the questions posed.

A 45-year-old has a clinical work-up, which included a nuclear medicine lung scan. The scan was positive, so chest images were ordered. The posteroanterior chest film is shown below.

A

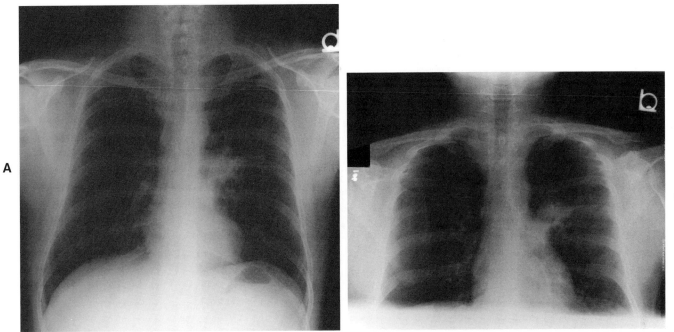

B

1. On image A, describe the area where the irregular radiopaque lesion is seen.

2. The area of interest needs to be better demonstrated, so what imaging could be used?

3. Before computerized tomography, conventional tomography was used to better delineate an anatomic structure or region. The slice thickness for tomographic imaging is controlled by what two factors?

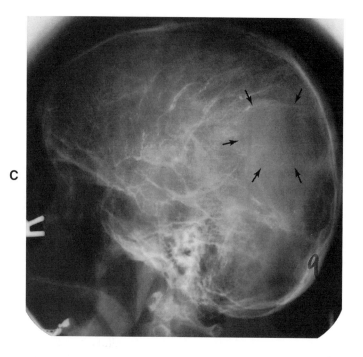

4. The patient was also experiencing headaches, so a cerebral angiogram was completed, as shown in

   image C. The arrows represent an encircling stain representative of a(n) _____
   [Hint: What pathology has an enhancing rim?].

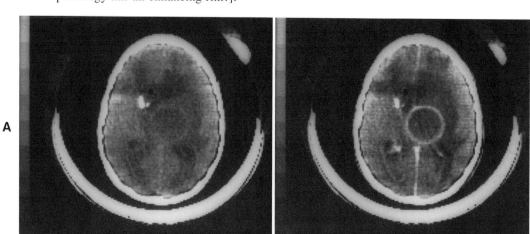

5. With the development of computerized technology, CT can demonstrate an abscess with better definition. On image A, the nonenhanced CT scan demonstrates a circular area with necrosis and possible
   liquefaction. On image B, the contrast enhanced CT scan, what does the same area appears as?

A 71-year-old with a history of hypertension, chronic renal insufficiency, rheumatoid arthritis, and known carotid artery disease was evaluated. On physical examination, a bulging area on the neck was noticed, which also pulsated.

1. An angiogram was completed to study which artery?

2. When plaque disease (atherosclerosis) is demonstrated, the patient will go to surgery to have what procedure?

3. Following the surgery, the patient had a color duplex Doppler ultrasound to evaluate the carotid artery. The scan was abnormal, so a follow-up carotid arteriogram was performed. Images A and B on the following page demonstrate an outpouching, which is suggestive of what?

123

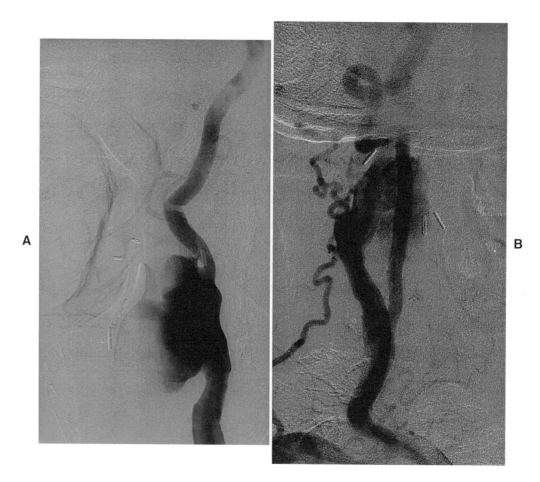

This patient's post-op arteriogram was positive for a pseudoaneurysm. The Doppler ultrasound measured the pseudo-aneurysm as 6 × 4 cm.

CASE STUDY 3

A young patient enters the emergency room with a severe headache. MRI demonstrates a mass of varying intensities caused by different blood flow rates in the region.

1. An irregular tangle of vessels and greatly dilated vessels is demonstrated. On images A and B on the following page, what is this anatomic disorder known as?

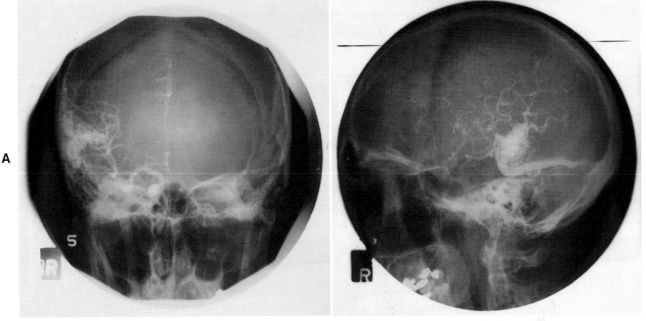

A

B

2. In this case, neurointervention was accomplished. Comparing image B with image C (below), why is the area of the malformation less visualized?

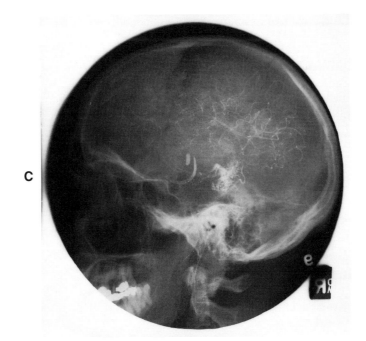

C

Detachable balloons were deployed to cause embolization. This saves the patient from undergoing surgery on the brain. There are still many risks involved; however, the recovery period for an interventional procedure is much less.

A 1-month-old baby is brought to the radiology department for a follow-up anteroposterior and lateral skull films.

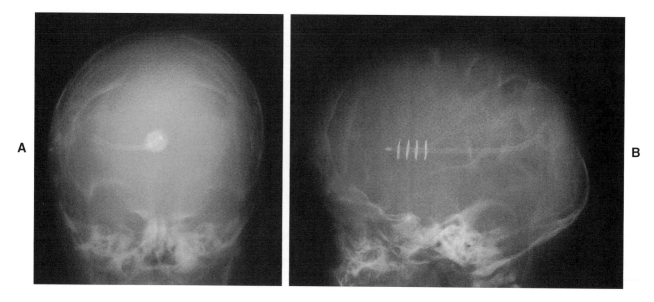

A   B

1. The inner table of the skull is uneven due to an increased internal fluid pressure. What is the name of the fluid?

2. What is the disorder of excessive fluid surrounding the brain tissue?

   What are the two types?

3. On the image, there appears to be an artifact. What does this artifact represent?

What is its purpose?

4. What imaging would best demonstrate the size of the fluid-filled spaces? Why?

This skull is said to have the lückenschädel appearance due to increased pressure from cerebrospinal fluid, as a result of hydrocephalus.

SELF-TEST

Read each question carefully, then circle the best answer.
1. A viral inflammation of the brain and meninges is called _____.
    a. meningitis
    b. hydrocephalus
    c. encephalitis
    d. encephalomalacia

2. The _____ space contains spinal fluid.
    a. subarachnoid
    b. epidural
    c. subdural
    d. epidermis

3. The imaging modality of choice to evaluate patients with suspected neurologic dysfunction caused by head trauma is _____.
    a. ultrasound
    b. MRI
    c. CT
    d. skull radiographs

4. A suppurative process in the space between the inner surface of the dura and the outer arachnoid surface is a(n)
    a. subdural empyema
    b. epidural empyema
    c. subarachnoid empyema
    d. brain abscess

5. A primary malignant tumor presenting a high signal intensity on T2-weighted MR images is a(n)
    a. chromophobe adenoma
    b. acoustic neuroma
    c. glioma
    d. pituitary adenoma

Chapter **8** **Nervous System**

6. A(n) _____ hematoma appears as a biconvex peripheral high-density lesion on CT.
   a. subdural
   b. epidural
   c. meningeal
   d. subarachnoid

7. Most _____ have calcifications, which can be visualized on routine skull images.
   a. meningioma
   b. craniopharyngioma
   c. glioma
   d. chromophobe adenoma

8. A linear skull fracture that intersects the sutures and continues along the sutures is a _____ fracture.
   a. diastatic
   b. tripod
   c. zygomatic
   d. blowout

9. Bleeding into the ventricular system as a result of injury to the surface veins is a(n) _____ hemorrhage.
   a. intracerebral
   b. subarachnoid
   c. intraparenchymal
   d. subdural

10. _____ refers to any process caused by an abnormality of the blood supply to the brain.
   a. Cerebrovascular accident
   b. Cerebrovascular disease
   c. Stroke syndrome
   d. Transient ischemic attack

11. A disease process seen as scattered plaque on MR images as a result of demyelination is
   a. Parkinson's disease
   b. multiple sclerosis
   c. Huntington's disease
   d. amyotrophic lateral sclerosis

12. Atrophy of the caudate nucleus and putamen seen on CT as focal dilatation of the frontal horns with a loss of their normal shape is indicative of
   a. amyotrophic lateral sclerosis
   b. Huntington's disease
   c. multiple sclerosis
   d. Parkinson's disease

13. The tumor that grows slowly, has an infiltrating character, and can form large cavities and pseudocysts is
   a. meningioma
   b. chordoma
   c. acoustic neuroma
   d. astrocytoma

14. The rim of low intensity consisting of a cerebrospinal fluid cleft, the vascular rim, or dura demonstrating separation of the tumor from adjacent brain, seen on T1- and T2-weighted MR images, is
    a. meningioma
    b. chordoma
    c. acoustic neuroma
    d. astrocytoma

15. A fracture of the zygomatic arch and the orbital floor, and a separation of the zygomaticofrontal suture is a(n) _____ fracture.
    a. Le Fort
    b. tripod
    c. blowout
    d. linear

16. A loculated infection most commonly seen in the gray matter is a(n)
    a. brain abscess
    b. bacterial meningitis
    c. subdural empyema
    d. encephalitis

17. Increased intracranial pressure caused by a blockage is suggestive of
    a. normal pressure hydrocephalus
    b. a grand mal seizure
    c. epilepsy
    d. noncommunicating hydrocephalus

18. A generalized convulsion that is associated with a patient falling, hypersalivation, and incontinence is considered
    a. epilepsy
    b. a grand mal seizure
    c. a petit mal seizure
    d. Parkinson's disease

19. Presenile progressive cerebral atrophy is _____ disease.
    a. Huntington's
    b. Lou Gehrig's
    c. Alzheimer's
    d. cerebrovascular

20. A berry aneurysm rupture is the major cause of a(n) _____ hemorrhage.
    a. intracerebral
    b. subdural
    c. epidural
    d. subarachnoid

9 Hematopoietic System

OBJECTIVES

In addition to the objectives listed at the beginning of Chapter 9 in the textbook, the user should be able to:

1. Identify anatomic structures on diagrams and radiographs of the hematopoietic system.
2. Describe the physiology of the hematopoietic system.
3. Differentiate the pathologic disorders of the hematopoietic system by defining the disease processes and their radiographic manifestations.
4. Determine changes in technical factors to obtain optimal-quality radiographs for patients with various underlying pathologic conditions.

EXERCISE 1—LABELING

A, The formed elements of blood.

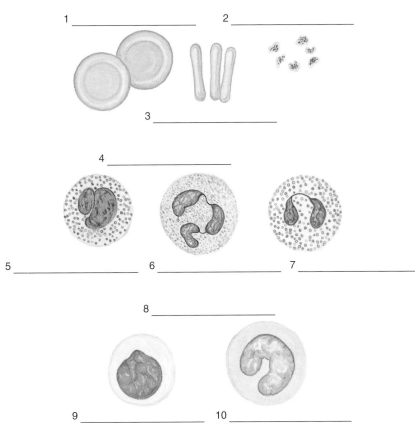

1 _____   2 _____

3 _____

4 _____

5 _____   6 _____   7 _____

8 _____

9 _____   10 _____

From Thibodeau GA, Patton KT: *Anatomy and physiology*, ed 6, St Louis, 2007, Mosby Elsevier.

Complete the following questions by writing the correct term(s) in the blank(s) provided.

1. Adequate blood supply brings what four necessary components to the cells?

   a. _____

   b. _____

   c. _____

   d. _____

2. Blood also provides a major defense system against

   a. _____

   b. _____

   c. _____

3. Blood-forming tissues in the body are

   a. _____

   b. _____

4. Red bone marrow makes which blood cells?

   a. _____

   b. _____

   c. _____

5. White blood cells are produced in the

   a. _____

   b. _____

6. Name the five types of leukocytes.

   a. _____

   b. _____

   c. _____

   d. _____

   e. _____

7. The _____ defends the body against bacteria by ingesting the foreign microorganisms and destroying them.

8. The smallest blood cell provides the essentials for blood clotting and is the _____.

132

EXERCISE 3—FILL IN THE BLANK: HEMATOPOIETIC PATHOLOGY

Complete the following questions by writing the correct term(s) in the blank(s) provided.

1. A decreased amount of oxygen-carrying hemoglobin is present in the peripheral blood as a result of

   _____.

2. Name three types of hemolytic anemias.

   a. _____

   b. _____

   c. _____

3. The fish vertebrae appearance occurs in _____ _____ anemia and is caused by indentations on the superior and inferior margins of soft vertebral bodies.

4. The "hair-on-end" appearance is vertical striations in a radial pattern due to _____.

5. _____ anemia is caused by a lack of vitamin B_{12} or folic acid.

6. Severe chronic pulmonary disease or congenital cyanotic heart disease causes long-term inadequate oxygen supplies

   in patients with _____ _____.

7. Due to cancer of the bone marrow, there is a huge increase in the number of circulating granulocytes and a decreased

   production of red blood cells and platelets in _____ _____.

8. A lymph node malignancy with a dramatic increase in lymphocytes is _____

   _____.

9. As the disease progresses, there may be bone destruction causing patchy lytic (moth-eaten) lesions to appear radio

   graphically in cases of _____.

10. Neoplasms of the lymphoreticular system are _____.

11. The lymphoreticular system includes

    a. _____

    b. _____

    c. _____

12. Ninety percent of all lymphoma cases are _____ _____.

13. Hodgkin's lymphoma originates in _____ _____ in most cases.

14. Parenchymal organs are the originating point for _____ _____.

15. The most common radiographic finding in lymphoma is lymph node enlargement in the

    _____, which is bilateral but asymmetric.

16. In lymphoma staging, _____ imaging can detect microscopic foci and alterations in function within normal-size nodes.

17. Epstein-Barr virus may cause _____.

18. Name the three components required for coagulation to occur.

   a. _____

   b. _____

   c. _____

19. _____ causes hemorrhages in the small bowel, producing a characteristic uniform regular thickening of mucosal folds in the bowel segment affected.

EXERCISE 4—MATCHING: ANATOMY AND PHYSIOLOGY

Match each of the following terms with the correct definition by placing the letter of the best answer in the space provided. Each question has only one correct answer. Please note that there are more terms than definitions.

1. _____ an iron-based protein that carries the oxygen from the lungs to the cells in the body

2. _____ biconcave disks without a nucleus that contain hemoglobin

3. _____ cell that plays a major role in the immune system and aids in the synthesis of antibodies

4. _____ contains granules that stain blue

5. _____ defends the body against bacteria

6. _____ red-staining cells that increase greatly in instances of allergy or parasitic conditions

7. _____ smallest blood cell essential for clotting

8. _____ supplies nutrients, oxygen, salt, and hormones to the cells and carries away waste products

A. basophil

B. blood

C. coagulation factors

D. eosinophil

E. erythrocytes (red)

F. hemoglobin

G. leukocytes

H. lymphocytes

I. monocytes

J. neutrophil

K. platelets

EXERCISE 5—MATCHING: HEMATOPOIETIC PATHOLOGY

Match each of the following terms with the correct definition by placing the letter of the best answer in the space provided. Each question has only one correct answer. Please note that there are more terms than definitions.

1. _____ anomaly of blood coagulation

2. _____ erythrocyte has an abnormal circular shape, making them vulnerable and susceptible to rupture

3. _____ generalized failure of the bone marrow function

4. _____ Hodgkin's and non-Hodgkin's

5. _____ hyperplasia of the bone marrow resulting in an increased production of red blood cells, granulocytes, and platelets

6. _____ neoplastic proliferation of white blood cells

7. _____ person appears pale due to lack of hemoglobin in the blood

8. _____ radiographically seen as a tubular bald stomach, reflecting a decrease or absence of the usual rugal folds

9. _____ red blood cells are crescent or sickle shaped and tend to rupture

10. _____ self-limited viral disease of the lymphoreticular system characterized by vague symptoms

11. _____ shortened red blood cell life span resulting in hemolysis

12. _____ spontaneous hemorrhages in the skin due to a deficiency in the number of platelets

A. anemia

B. aplastic anemia

C. hemolytic anemia

D. hemophilia

E. infectious mononucleosis

F. leukemia

G. lymphoma

H. megaloblastic anemia

I. myelocytic leukemia

J. pernicious anemia

K. polycythemia (primary)

L. purpura

M. sickle cell anemia

N. spherocytosis

O. thalassemia

EXERCISE 6—MULTIPLE CHOICE

Circle the best answer for the following multiple choice questions.

1. A decrease in the amount of oxygen-carrying hemoglobin in the peripheral blood is
   a. polycythemia
   b. leukemia
   c. anemia
   d. lymphoma

2. Spherocytosis, sickle cell anemia, and thalassemia are examples of _____ anemias.
   a. iron deficiency
   b. hemolytic
   c. pernicious
   d. myelophthisic

3. Cortical thinning with pronounced widening of the medullary cavity is suggestive of
   a. thalassemia
   b. megaloblastic anemia
   c. sickle cell anemia
   d. iron deficiency anemia

4. Gastric atrophy seen radiographically as a stomach with a bald appearance (lack of rugal folds) may indicate
   a. pernicious anemia
   b. sickle cell anemia
   c. polycythemia
   d. thalassemia

5. In sickle cell anemia, the red blood cells are
   a. crescent shaped
   b. circular and fragile
   c. biconcave
   d. not carrying oxygen

6. Aplastic anemia results in
   a. vitamin B_{12} deficiency
   b. decreased levels of erythrocytes and platelets
   c. decreased red and white blood cells
   d. hyperplasia of the bone marrow

7. Cancer of the bone marrow causing proliferation of white blood cells is
   a. lymphatic leukemia
   b. lymphoma
   c. polycythemia
   d. myelocytic leukemia

8. The most common radiographic finding in lymphoma is
   a. mediastinal lymph node enlargement
   b. splenomegaly
   c. prominent pulmonary vascular shadows
   d. localized steplike central depressions of the vertebra

9. In cases of lymphoma, the best modality to demonstrate microscopic tumor foci is
   a. computed tomography (CT)
   b. magnetic resonance imaging
   c. nuclear medicine
   d. positron emission tomography

10. A lifelong tendency for spontaneous hemorrhage is
    a. hemolytic anemia
    b. mononucleosis
    c. hemophilia
    d. purpura

EXERCISE 7—CASE STUDY

The following is a case study in which pelvic imaging was requested. In this scenario, you will see the images and be asked to answer questions. Using the knowledge of imaging pathology, apply exposure factors and positioning criteria to answer the questions posed.

A male patient born in 1957 was diagnosed with Hodgkin's lymphoma. The patient underwent therapy and was doing well. Currently the patient is experiencing mid and lower abdominal pain, so follow-up scans of the abdomen and pelvis were ordered.

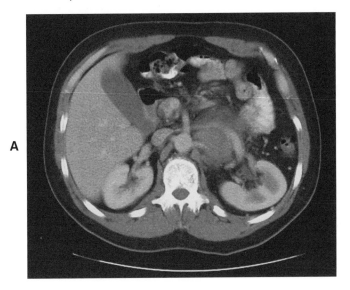

A

1. Differentiate Hodgkin's and non-Hodgkin's lymphoma.

2. Which modalities are most useful in staging and treatment follow up?

The conglomerate lymph nodal mass is displacing the renal vein anteriorly.

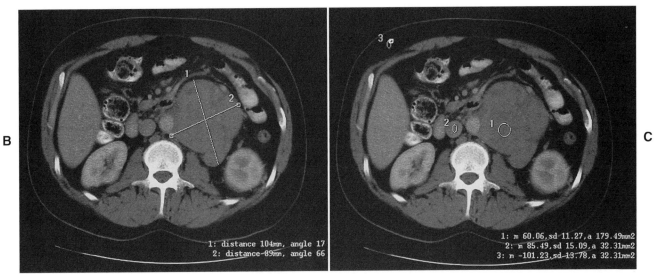

B

1: distance 104mm, angle 17
2: distance 89mm, angle 66

1: m 60.06,sd 11.27,a 179.49mm2
2: m 85.49,sd 15.09,a 32.31mm2
3: m -101.23,sd 13.78,a 32.31mm2

C

137

3. Referring to the image, what does the mass measures?

4. Three regions of interest (ROI) were recorded. What CT numbers are derived?

5. In which ROI is the CT number closest to the value of water?

6. Fat has a CT number less than 0. Which ROI would this be?

SELF-TEST

Read each question carefully, then circle the best answer.
1. When diseases of the hematopoietic system result in demineralization of bone, the radiographer must be alert to
   a. patient infection
   b. pathologic fracture
   c. self-infection
   d. parasites

2. White blood cells
   a. are the smallest blood cell and are required for clotting
   b. aid in the immune system and aid in antibody synthesis
   c. carry hemoglobin
   d. are an iron-based protein carrying oxygen

3. Which term refers to a decrease in the amount of oxygen-carrying hemoglobin in the blood?
   a. thalassemia
   b. erythrocytosis
   c. anemia
   d. thrombocytopenia

4. Erythrocytes have an abnormal circular shape, which makes them vulnerable and susceptible to rupture in cases of
   a. thalassemia
   b. megaloblastic anemia
   c. thrombocytopenia
   d. spherocytosis

138

5. Thalassemia radiographically presents as
   a. pronounced medullary cavity widening and cortical thinning
   b. localized steplike central depressions of the vertebra
   c. cardiomegaly
   d. gastric atrophy

6. Spontaneous hemorrhages in the skin caused by a lack of platelets is
   a. hemophilia
   b. infectious mononucleosis
   c. purpura
   d. polycythemia

7. The anemia most often seen in blacks, in which red cells are crescentic and tend to rupture, is
   a. sickle cell anemia
   b. thalassemia
   c. lymphoma
   d. thrombocytopenia

8. Abnormalities in blood coagulation is known as
   a. hemophilia
   b. aplastic anemia
   c. thrombocytopenia
   d. purpura

9. Aplastic anemia is associated with
   a. folic acid deficiency, causing loss of DNA synthesis
   b. generalized bone marrow failure
   c. proliferation of white blood cells
   d. neoplastic growths of the lymphoreticular system

10. The shortened life span of red blood cells is characteristic of _____ anemia.
   a. hemolytic
   b. iron deficiency
   c. megaloblastic
   d. pernicious

10 Endocrine System

In addition to the objectives listed at the beginning of Chapter 10 in the textbook, the user should be able to:
1. Identify anatomic structures on diagrams and radiographs of the endocrine system.
2. Describe the physiology of the endocrine system.
3. Differentiate the pathologic disorders of the endocrine system by defining the disease processes and their radiographic manifestations.
4. Determine changes in technical factors to obtain optimal-quality radiographs for patients with various underlying pathologic conditions.

EXERCISE 1—LABELING: ANATOMY

A, Adrenal gland.

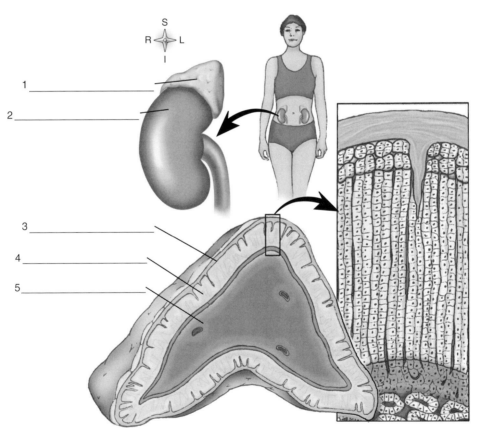

From Thibodeau GA, Patton KT: *Anatomy and physiology*, ed 6, St Louis, 2007, Mosby Elsevier.

B, Pituitary and hormones.

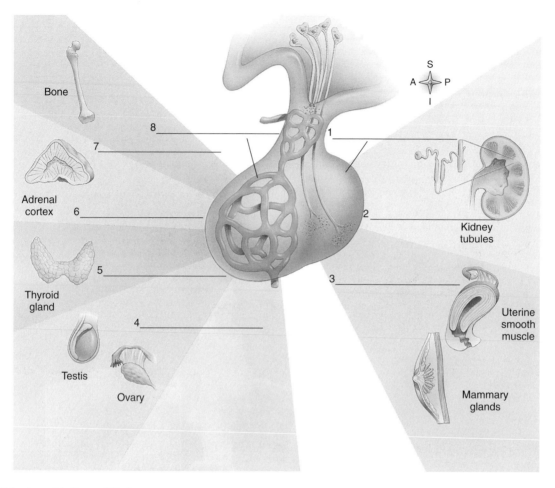

Bone

8 _____

7 _____

Adrenal
cortex   6 _____

Thyroid
gland   5 _____

4 _____

Testis

Ovary

S
A ⟷ P
I

1 _____

2 _____
Kidney
tubules

3 _____
Uterine
smooth
muscle

Mammary
glands

From Thibodeau GA, Patton KT: *Anatomy and physiology*, ed 6, St Louis, 2007, Mosby Elsevier.

Chapter **10   Endocrine System**

C, Thyroid and parathyroid glands.

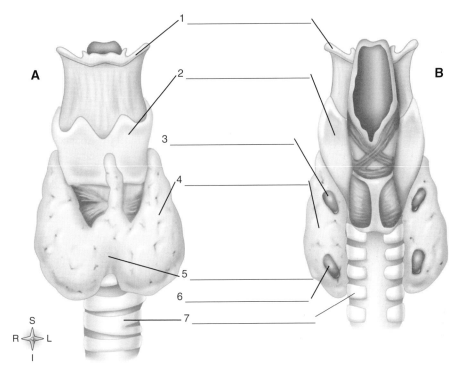

1 _____

2 _____

3 _____

4 _____

5 _____

6 _____

7 _____

A   B

S
R ←✦→ L
I

A, From Jacob: *Atlas of human anatomy,* 2002, Elsevier. **B,** From Thibodeau GA, Patton KT: *Anatomy and physiology,* ed 6, St Louis, 2007, Mosby Elsevier.

EXERCISE 2—FILL IN THE BLANK: ANATOMY AND PHYSIOLOGY

Complete the following questions by writing the correct term(s) in the blank(s) provided.

1. The _____ _____ is situated on top of the kidney and each component secretes different hormones.

2. _____ regulate salt and water balance by controlling kidney excretions of potassium and sodium retention.

3. Glucocorticoids regulate _____ _____.

4. Androgens are sex hormones that

   a. _____

   b. _____

   c. _____

5. The adrenal medulla secretes _____ and _____.

6. The hormonal secretions of the pituitary gland are controlled by the _____.

7. The pituitary gland sits in the bony depression in the spheroid bone called the _____

   _____.

143

8. Growth hormone (GH) promotes _____ growth and _____ of the tissues.

9. Oxytocin is secreted by the _____ pituitary gland and causes contraction of _____ _____.

10. In response to the body's need for increased energy production, _____ stimulates cellular metabolism.

11. The _____ _____ is a butterfly-shaped gland consisting of two lobes.

12. The _____ _____ are the glands responsible for controlling levels of blood calcium and phosphate.

13. Parathormone increases a low calcium level by what three mechanisms?

    a. _____

    b. _____

    c. _____

14. _____ _____ is a common endocrine disorder when beta cells in the islets of Langerhans fail to secrete insulin.

EXERCISE 3—FILL IN THE BLANK: ENDOCRINE SYSTEM PATHOLOGY

Complete the following questions by writing the correct term(s) in the blank(s) provided.

1. Nontumorous hyperfunction is most often the cause of _____ _____.

2. The most superficial layer of the adrenal cortex causes retention of sodium and water and an abnormal loss of potassium in the urine in cases of _____.

3. Elevated levels of androgens cause accelerated skeletal maturation along with premature epiphyseal fusion in _____ syndrome.

4. A typical higher signal intensity is seen on T2-weighted images in _____ metastasis demonstrating contrast enhancement.

5. Pheochromocytomas can be diagnosed with _____ _____; imaging aids only in confirmation.

6. About 50% of these tumors have calcifications, which distinguish them from Wilms' tumor; these represent _____.

7. Gigantism and acromegaly are examples of _____.

8. An excessively large skeleton is a manifestation of _____.

9. _____ causes profound generalized disturbances in bone growth and maturation.

10. Severe polyuria leads to massive dilatation of the renal pelves, calyces, and ureters in _____

_____.

11. The modality of choice to determine the function of the thyroid for both palpable and nonpalpable nodules is

_____ _____.

12. A solid mass with a consistent echogenicity, often demonstrating a thick smooth periphery of a capsule, is a

_____ _____ _____.

13. Name three types of thyroid carcinoma.

   a. _____

   b. _____

   c. _____

14. Name the three categories of hyperparathyroidism.

   a. _____

   b. _____

   c. _____

15. _____ _____ produces a variety of radiographic findings involving
multiple systems, including atherosclerosis, susceptible to infection and neuropathy.

Match each of the following terms with the correct definition by placing the letter of the best answer in the space provided. Each question has only one correct answer. Please note that there are more terms than definitions.

1. _____ butterfly-shaped gland located in the neck

2. _____ control sodium retention and potassium secretion

3. _____ four tiny glands on the superior and inferior posterior aspects of the thyroid gland

4. _____ increase rate of absorption of water and electrolytes by renal tubules

5. _____ inner medulla and outer cortex

6. _____ natural iodine-containing substance to stimulate cellular metabolism

7. _____ produces two hormones: vasopressin and oxytocin

8. _____ promotes growth and development of all parts of the body

9. _____ regulates carbohydrate metabolism

10. _____ regulation of the menstrual cycle and secretion of sex hormones (male and female)

11. _____ responsible for controlling calcium and phosphate blood levels

12. _____ secretes a group of hormones affecting the sex organs or gonads

13. _____ sex hormones

14. _____ stimulates heart activity and raises blood pressure

15. _____ the master gland controlled by the hypothalamus

A. adrenal glands

B. androgens

C. anterior lobe of pituitary gland

D. epinephrine

E. glucocorticoids

F. gonadotropin

G. growth hormone

H. hyperactive endocrine glands

I. luteinizing hormone

J. mineralocorticoids

K. oxytocin

L. parathormone

M. parathyroid glands

N. pituitary gland

O. posterior lobe of pituitary gland

P. thyroid gland

Q. thyroxine

R. vasopressin

Match each of the following terms with the correct definition by placing the letter of the best answer in the space provided. Each question has only one correct answer. Please note that there are more terms than definitions.

1. _____ a lack of insulin prevents glucose from entering cells

2. _____ characteristic obesity of the body's trunk and a moon-shaped face

3. _____ due to overproduction of hormones, hypertension, muscular weakness, and excessive thirst are the results

4. _____ encapsulated mass usually compressing adjacent tissue

5. _____ enlargement of the thyroid gland not causing inflammation or neoplasia

6. _____ excessive growth hormone produced by a tumor

7. _____ excessive production of thyroxine

8. _____ exists in the adrenal medulla and produces excess vasopressors

9. _____ failure of normal end-organ response to normal levels of circulating hormones

10. _____ functional abnormality leading to an insufficient synthesis of thyroid hormone

11. _____ generalized disorder of calcium, phosphate, and bone metabolism

12. _____ kidneys' inability to conserve water, resulting in low blood levels of ADH (antidiuretic hormone)

13. _____ loss of secretion of any anterior pituitary hormone

14. _____ pulmonary, breast, renal, and ovarian carcinomas most frequently spread here

15. _____ most cases are caused by adrenocortical tumors

16. _____ papillary, follicular, and medullary are types of this neoplasia

17. _____ predominantly affects females symptomatically as nervousness, emotional liability, and inability to sleep

18. _____ rapidly growing mass usually necrotic at the time of clinical presentation

19. _____ symptoms are fatigue, anorexia, weakness, weight loss, hypotension, vomiting, and diarrhea

20. _____ ultrasound is the modality of choice to evaluate this abdominal mass in children

A. acromegaly

B. adrenal carcinoma

C. adrenal metastases

D. adrenogenital syndrome

E. aldosteronism

F. benign thyroid adenoma

G. Cushing's syndrome

H. diabetes insipidus

I. diabetes mellitus

J. goiter

K. Graves' disease

L. hyperglycemia

M. hyperparathyroidism

N. hyperpituitarism

O. hyperthyroidism

P. hypoadrenalism

Q. hypoparathyroidism

R. hypopituitarism

S. hypothyroidism

T. neuroblastoma

U. pheochromocytoma

V. pseudohypoparathyroidism

W. thyroid carcinoma

Circle the best answer for the following multiple choice questions.

1. Computed tomography (CT) is the modality of choice to evaluate for _____ because of the radiographic changes produced in multiple systems.
   a. aldosteronism
   b. adrenogenital syndrome
   c. Cushing's syndrome
   d. hypoadrenalism

2. In cases of _____, the role of imaging is to demonstrate the location of the adenoma, which will be difficult to detect during surgery.
   a. aldosteronism
   b. hypoadrenalism
   c. adrenal virilism
   d. Addison's disease

3. Excessive administration of steroids is the most common cause of
   a. aldosteronism
   b. hyperadrenalism
   c. adrenogenital syndrome
   d. hypoadrenalism

4. Adrenal carcinomas are best demonstrated on
   a. CT as a large irregular edged mass
   b. US as a complex mass, which is difficult to separate from the kidney
   c. Magnetic resonance imaging (MRI) as an inflammatory process causing enlargement
   d. General x-rays, a kidney-ureter-bladder image

5. Arterial injections of iodinated contrast agents cause a sharp elevation in blood pressure for patients with
   a. neuroblastoma
   b. pheochromocytoma
   c. adrenal carcinoma
   d. adrenal metastasis

6. Thickened bones of the skull, enlarged paranasal sinuses, and lengthened mandible are all suggestive of
   a. hypopituitarism
   b. acromegaly
   c. hyperpituitarism
   d. hyperthyroidism

7. The gland that controls the level of secretion of gonadal and thyroid hormones and the production of GH is the _____ gland.
   a. adrenal
   b. pituitary
   c. thyroid
   d. parathyroid

8. MRI is the modality of choice to demonstrate a pituitary tumor because of the
   a. multiplanar imaging abilities
   b. tumor size
   c. tumor location
   d. all of the above

9. Uniform radioactivity throughout the thyroid that demonstrates diffuse enlargement is suggestive of
   a. Addison's disease
   b. Graves' disease
   c. Conn's syndrome
   d. Cushing's syndrome

10. In severe cases of Graves' disease, the patient may have associated
    a. skeletal overgrowth and bone spurs
    b. generalized cardiomegaly and pulmonary congestion
    c. complex masses with an irregular periphery
    d. none of the above

11. An enlargement of the thyroid gland that is not inflammatory or neoplastic is
    a. a goiter
    b. an adenoma
    c. Graves' disease
    d. Addison's disease

12. The most common type of thyroid carcinoma is
    a. papillary
    b. medullary
    c. follicular
    d. cortical

13. Spreading to regional lymph nodes, _____ is slow growing and cystic.
    a. medullary carcinoma
    b. papillary carcinoma
    c. neuroblastoma
    d. pheochromocytoma

14. The thyroid carcinoma that closely mimics normal thyroid tissue is the _____ type.
    a. follicular
    b. adenomatous
    c. medullary
    d. stem cell

15. Common manifestations of diabetes mellitus are
    a. polyuria, dysphagia, and hyperglycemia
    b. hyperglycemia, adenopathy, and polydipsia
    c. polyuria, polydipsia, and glycosuria
    d. hypoglycemic shock, polydipsia, and glycosuria

SELF-TEST

Read each question carefully, then circle the best answer.

1. The endocrine system controls
   a. a broad range of vital body activities
   b. a communication network through several glands
   c. secretion of chemical messengers
   d. all of the above

2. The hormones regulating carbohydrate metabolism are
   a. glucocorticoids
   b. androgens
   c. mineralocorticoids
   d. gonadotropins

3. Generalized enlargement of the adrenal glands is best demonstrated by
   a. ultrasound appearing anechoic
   b. CT appearing as thickened wings
   c. MRI as a functioning microadenoma
   d. none of the above

4. An abnormal loss of potassium in the urine can be caused by a(n)
   a. overproduction of mineralocorticoid hormones
   b. excessive amount of androgens
   c. abundance of glucocorticoids
   d. loss of androgens

5. The adrenal gland producing excessive androgenic active hormones causes
   a. Addison's disease
   b. Graves' disease
   c. Conn's syndrome
   d. adrenogenital syndrome

6. The most common cause of hypoadrenalism is
   a. steroid administration
   b. excessive mineralocorticoids
   c. excessive glucose
   d. excessive insulin

7. Lymphatic and hepatic metastasis is common when _____ presents clinically because of rapid growth (usually necrotic).
   a. adrenal carcinoma
   b. neuroblastoma
   c. pheochromocytoma
   d. thyroid carcinoma

8. The most common carcinomas to metastasize to the adrenal gland are
   a. lung and prostate cancers
   b. breast and prostate cancers
   c. lung and breast cancers
   d. lung and brain cancers

9. The tumor that produces an excessive amount of vasopressor substances is a(n)
   a. adrenal carcinoma
   b. pheochromocytoma
   c. neuroblastoma
   d. aldosteronism

10. Calcifications in a _____ have a fine granular or stippled appearance.
    a. pheochromocytoma
    b. neuroblastoma
    c. adrenal metastases
    d. thyroid goiter

11. The modality of choice to diagnose a neuroblastoma is
    a. CT
    b. ultrasound
    c. MRI
    d. nuclear medicine

12. The posterior lobe of the pituitary gland produces
    a. vasopressin and epinephrine
    b. oxytocin and norepinephrine
    c. vasopressin and oxytocin
    d. epinephrine and norepinephrine

13. Hyperpituitarism after bone growth stops causes
    a. gigantism
    b. elephantiasis
    c. acromegaly
    d. edema

14. Radiographers need to be cautious of complications of Cushing's syndrome, such as
    a. sella erosion
    b. hypercalciuria
    c. spontaneous fractures
    d. frequent infections

15. These hormones are known as fight or flight; they are
    a. androgen and adrenaline
    b. epinephrine and adrenaline
    c. glucocorticoid and androgen
    d. epinephrine and norepinephrine

16. The modality that demonstrates function of the thyroid gland the best is
    a. ultrasound
    b. CT
    c. nuclear medicine
    d. MRI

150

17. Graves' disease results from an excessive production of thyroid hormone known as
    a. hyperparathyroidism
    b. hyperpituitarism
    c. hyperthyroidism
    d. hypopituitarism

18. Cretinism, which usually results in short stature, is considered the result of an abnormality of an insufficient synthesis of thyroid hormone known as
    a. hypothyroidism
    b. hypopituitarism
    c. hypoparathyroidism
    d. Addison's disease

19. Thyroid adenomas appear "hot" or "cold" on nuclear medicine scans depending upon their
    a. functional capacity
    b. anatomic location
    c. interaction
    d. physiology

20. The thyroid carcinoma peaking in young adulthood and again in the third and fifth decades and that is slow growing is
    a. papillary carcinoma
    b. medullary carcinoma
    c. follicular carcinoma
    d. adenocarcinoma

21. Diabetes mellitus is a result of the
    a. pancreas failing to secrete insulin
    b. pancreas producing excessive insulin
    c. kidneys conserving water
    d. kidneys' failure to conserve water

22. Sustained muscular contraction due to a lack of parathormone is
    a. hypothyroidism
    b. hypoparathyroidism
    c. pseudohypoparathyroidism
    d. hypopituitarism

23. The parathyroid disease process often attributed to chronic renal failure is
    a. primary hyperparathyroidism
    b. secondary hyperparathyroidism
    c. tertiary hyperparathyroidism
    d. follicular hyperparathyroidism

24. On ultrasound, these tumors generally appear as solid hypoechoic masses and may contain microcalcifications; they are
    a. papillary carcinomas
    b. follicular carcinomas
    c. neuroblastomas
    d. pheochromocytomas

11 Reproductive System

OBJECTIVES

In addition to the objectives listed at the beginning of Chapter 11 in the textbook, the user should be able to:

1. Identify anatomic structures on diagrams and radiographs of the reproductive system.
2. Describe the physiology of the reproductive system.
3. Differentiate the pathologic disorders of the reproductive system by defining the disease processes and their radiographic manifestations.
4. Determine changes in technical factors to obtain optimal-quality radiographs for patients with various underlying pathologic conditions.

EXERCISE 1—LABELING: ANATOMY

Identify the anatomic structures indicated by writing the correct name in the space provided.

A, The male reproductive system.

14 _____

Ampulla
of ductus
deferens

1 _____

2 _____

3 _____

4 _____

Corpus
cavernosum

Corpus
spongiosum

13 _____

12 _____

11 _____

10 _____

9 _____

5 _____

S
R ✦ L
I

Glans
penis

8 _____

6 _____

7 _____

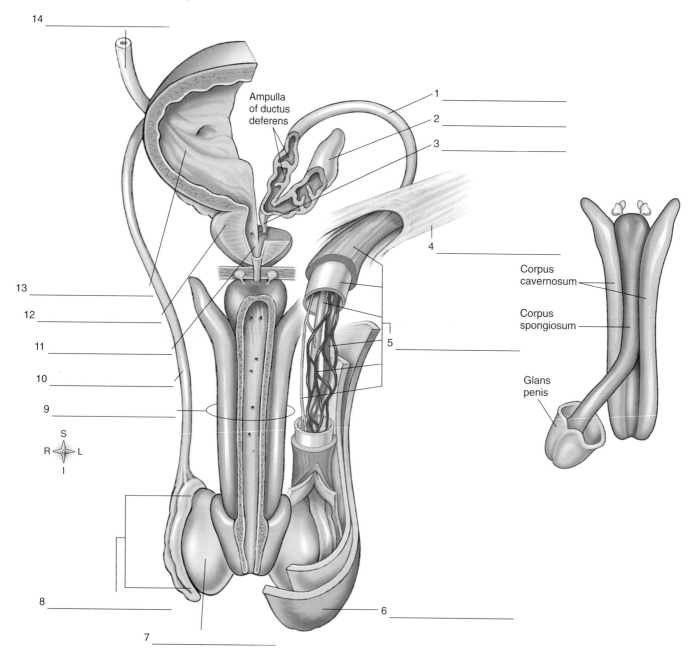

B, The female reproductive system.

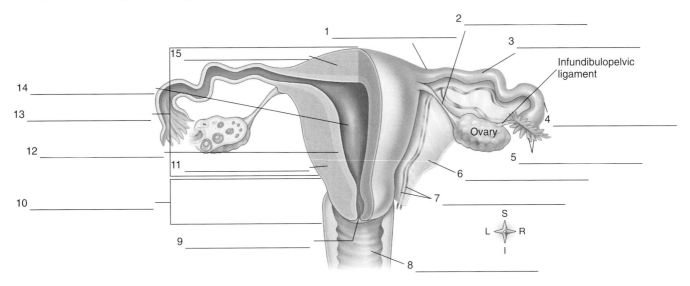

2 _____

1 _____

3 _____

15 _____

Infundibulopelvic ligament

14 _____

13 _____

Ovary

4 _____

12 _____

5 _____

11 _____

6 _____

7 _____

S

L ✦ R

I

10 _____

9 _____

8 _____

C, The female breast.

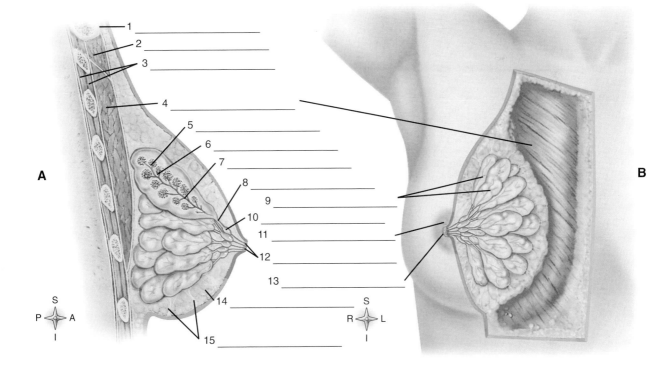

1 _____

2 _____

3 _____

4 _____

5 _____

6 _____

7 _____

8 _____

9 _____

10 _____

11 _____

12 _____

13 _____

14 _____

15 _____

A

B

S

P ✦ A

I

S

R ✦ L

I

Chapter **11** **Reproductive System**

Complete the following questions by writing the correct term(s) in the blank(s) provided.

1. The major function of the male reproductive system is the _____ of _____ (spermatogenesis).

2. Male germ cells are called _____.

3. Which endocrine gland stimulates the testes to produce germ cells? _____

4. The testes produce germ cells and secrete the male hormone _____.

5. The final maturation of the sperm occurs in the _____.

6. A muscular tube connecting the epididymis and that is part of the spermatic cord is the _____.

7. The _____ _____ and the vas deferens form the ejaculatory duct.

8. Severing the vas deferens to make the male sterile is a _____.

9. This structure lies on the posterior aspect at the base of the bladder and also secretes a thick liquid consisting of fructose. This structure is known as the _____ _____.

10. Male fertility is dependent upon

    a. _____

    b. _____

    c. _____

    d. _____

11. _____ refers to the onset of menstruation in females.

12. Ova begin to grow and develop to a mature ovum; this process of expelling the mature ovum is known as _____.

13. The corpus luteum continues to grow after the ovum has been released and secretes _____.

14. The ovum travels from the ovary to the uterus via the _____ _____.

15. Implantation of the fertilized ovum outside of the uterus is a(n) _____.

16. The _____ phase occurs between the end of menses and ovulation.

17. The phase of the menstrual cycle between ovulation and the onset of menses is _____.

18. The menstrual phase of the cycle is a result of what three products?

   a. _____

   b. _____

   c. _____

19. Natural termination of the reproductive processes is _____.

20. Surgical removal of the female reproductive organs is a _____.

EXERCISE 3—FILL IN THE BLANK: REPRODUCTIVE PATHOLOGY

Complete the following questions by writing the correct term(s) in the blank(s) provided.

1. In the secondary stage of syphilis, a _____ _____ affects any part of the body.

2. _____ can cause septic arthritis (joint erosion and narrowing).

3. Radiographically, the bladder on excretory urography is elevated by a smooth impression caused by

   _____ _____ _____.

4. To best delineate the prostate, seminal vesicles, and surrounding organs for accurate staging of carcinoma of the

   prostate gland, _____ is the modality of choice.

5. Inflammation of the pair (or one) of the long tightly coiled ducts that carry sperm from the seminiferous tubules

   of the testis(es) to the vas deferens is _____.

6. On ultrasound, a testicular tumor that has a uniform hypoechoic mass appearance without calcification or cystic

   areas is known as a _____.

7. Spread of infection into the fallopian tubes from the pelvis is caused by _____

   _____ _____.

8. As a result of pelvic inflammatory disease, the fallopian tubes may be obstructed, causing

   _____ or _____ _____.

9. Lipid material within the lesion with relative radiolucency that has a characteristic of calcification is a

   _____ _____.

10. Often multiple benign smooth-muscle tumors of the uterus, _____

   _____, are stimulated by estrogen.

11. Post menopausal bleeding is a symptom of _____ _____, which is
   the predominant neoplasm of the uterine body.

12. Endometrial tissue outside the uterus undergoes a proliferation and secretory phase because it responds to

   _____ _____.

13. The _____ _____ examination has permitted early detection of cervical carcinomas.

14. A tumor mass with clustered calcification in the mammory gland is indicative of _____

_____.

15. The most common benign breast tumor is a _____.

16. Fetal age is best demonstrated by _____.

17. Maternal disorders, such as diabetes mellitus and Rh isoimmunization, may cause _____ during pregnancy.

18. Most ectopic pregnancies occur in the _____ _____.

19. Abnormal fertilization that lacks the female chromosome is a _____.

20. The frequently malignant _____ is a primary tumor that develops from the chorionic portion of the products of conception.

EXERCISE 4—MATCHING: ANATOMY AND PHYSIOLOGY

Match each of the following terms with the correct definition by placing the letter of the best answer in the space provided. Each question has only one correct answer. Please note that there are more terms than definitions.

1. _____ duct for ova to reach uterus

2. _____ female reproductive life begins

3. _____ fertilization of ova outside the uterus

4. _____ final maturation of sperm occurs

5. _____ flow of blood, mucus, and sloughed endometrium

6. _____ formation of sperm

7. _____ male germ cells

8. _____ muscular tube passing through the inguinal canal

9. _____ ova mature and are expelled from the ovary

10. _____ produces major portion of the seminal fluid

11. _____ secrete a thick fluid of fructose

12. _____ testes secrete a male hormone

A. corpus luteum

B. ectopic pregnancy

C. ejaculatory duct

D. epididymis

E. fallopian tube

F. menarche

G. menstrual phase

H. ovulation

I. proliferative phase

J. prostate gland

K. seminal vesicles

L. spermatogenesis

M. spermatozoa

N. testosterone

O. vas deferens

Match each of the following terms with the correct definition by placing the letter of the best answer in the space provided. Each question has only one correct answer. Please note that there are more terms than definitions.

1. _____ arises from a primitive germ cell and consists of many tissue types

2. _____ benign ovarian tumor

3. _____ benign smooth-muscle tumor

4. _____ caused by spirochete *Treponema pallidum*

5. _____ causing an inability to empty the bladder completely

6. _____ ectopic testis

7. _____ elevated prostate-specific antigen, and a hard nodular and irregular mass on rectal exam

8. _____ excessive accumulation of amniotic fluid

9. _____ fallopian tube filled with pus

10. _____ fetal implantation outside of the uterus

11. _____ fibrocystic disease—cysts of various sizes distributed throughout the organ

12. _____ follicular and corpus luteum are examples

13. _____ germ cell tumor of ovary

14. _____ infection of the uterus and fallopian tubes

15. _____ most common and widely spread venereal disease

16. _____ most common malignancy in women

17. _____ neoplasm of the uterine body and most common invasive neoplasm

18. _____ normal-appearing endometrium in sites other than their normal location

19. _____ spectrum of diseases, including hydatidiform and choriocarcinoma

20. _____ tumor arising from the seminiferous tubules

21. _____ tumor related to chronic irritation, infection, and poor hygiene

22. _____ twisting of the gonad on its pedicle

23. _____ very small volume of amniotic fluid

A. benign breast disease

B. benign prostatic hyperplasia

C. breast cancer

D. carcinoma of the prostate gland

E. cervical carcinoma

F. cryptorchidism

G. cystadenoma

H. dermoid cyst

I. ectopic pregnancy

J. endometrial carcinoma

K. endometriosis

L. epididymitis

M. fibroadenoma

N. gonorrhea

O. infertility

P. oligohydramnios

Q. ovarian cysts

R. pelvic inflammatory disease

S. polyhydramnios

T. pyosalpinx

U. seminoma

V. syphilis

W. teratoma

X. testicular torsion

Y. trophoblastic disease

Z. uterine fibroids

Circle the best answer for the following multiple choice questions.

1. On magnetic resonance imaging (MRI), benign prostatic hyperplasia appears as
   a. homogeneous low signal on T1-weighted images
   b. heterogeneous high signal on T2-weighted images
   c. normal uniform high signal intensity
   d. inhomogeneous with cystic and solid areas

2. Prostate gland carcinoma impresses on the bladder as a
   a. smooth contour with elevation
   b. irregular contour with elevation
   c. thickened bladder wall
   d. irregular contour without elevation

3. The testis normally migrates through the _____ into the scrotal sac.
   a. perineal region
   b. levator ani muscle
   c. inguinal canal
   d. cremaster muscle

4. A compromise of circulation to the testis with sudden onset of severe scrotal pain is
   a. epididymitis
   b. cryptorchidism
   c. testicular agenesis
   d. testicular torsion

5. The modality of choice to demonstrate testicular tumors is
   a. computed tomography (CT)
   b. ultrasound
   c. MRI
   d. nuclear medicine

6. Abscesses with a thick irregular wall containing echoes on pelvic ultrasound images are suggestive of
   a. pyosalpinx
   b. hydrosalpinx
   c. pelvic inflammatory disease
   d. polycystic ovarian disease

7. On an abdominal x-ray, psammomatous calcifications appear as scattered, fine amorphous shadows (that are similar to normal soft tissue and easily missed) represent a
   a. cystadenoma
   b. ovarian cyst
   c. ovarian carcinoma
   d. cystadenocarcinoma

8. A cyst (ovarian) that has no clinical significance and is composed of germ cells, such as skin, hair, and teeth, is known as a(n)
   a. polycystic ovarian disease
   b. dermoid cyst
   c. cyst adenoma
   d. ovarian cyst

9. A poorly defined mass with irregular margins and numerous fine linear strands or spicules radiating out is indicative of
   a. fibrocystic disease
   b. breast cancer
   c. benign breast disease
   d. a fibroadenoma

10. A reflux of endometrial fragments backward through the fallopian tubes during menstruation, resulting in an implantation in the pelvis, is
    a. endometriosis
    b. ectopic pregnancy
    c. trophoblastic disease
    d. pelvic inflammatory disease

11. An enlarged uterus with irregular areas of low-level echoes and bizarre clusters of high-intensity echoes is suggestive of
    a. cervical carcinoma
    b. leiomyomas
    c. ovarian cysts
    d. endometrial carcinoma

12. A benign breast disease demonstrating various sized cysts throughout the breasts is
    a. fibrocystic disease
    b. cystoadenoma
    c. trophoblastic disease
    d. polycystic disease

13. A condition of pregnancy primarily resulting from fetal urinary disorders, such as renal dysplasia and renal aplasia, is
    a. polyhydramnios
    b. endometriosis
    c. trophoblastic disease
    d. oligohydramnios

14. An enlarged uterus that does not contain a gestational sac and that is associated with fluid in the cul-de-sac is suggestive of
    a. hydatidiform mole
    b. ectopic pregnancy
    c. choriocarcinoma
    d. endometriosis

15. Anomalies in the reproductive organs, obstructed fallopian tubes, and production of immature ova can cause
    a. pelvic inflammatory disease
    b. trophoblastic disease
    c. infertility
    d. leiomyomas

EXERCISE 7—CASE STUDY

The following is a case study in which abdominal imaging was requested. In this scenario, you will see an image and be asked to answer questions. Using the knowledge of imaging pathology, apply exposure factors and positioning criteria to answer the questions posed.

CASE STUDY 1

A female patient enters radiology with continued symptoms of pelvic cramping. A kidney-ureter-bladder (KUB) is performed and is shown below.

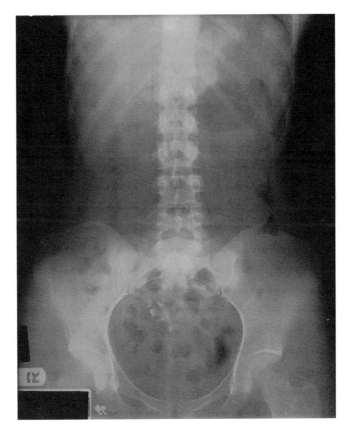

1. What anatomy is a KUB required to include?

2. How is the appropriate contrast in screen-film imaging accomplished?

3. Are there any abnormal structures seen?

   Where are they located?

4. Differential diagnosis?

SELF-TEST

Read each question carefully, then circle the best answer.

1. The tertiary stage of syphilis
   a. is treated with antibiotics
   b. causes multisystemic involvement
   c. results in skin lesions and a rash
   d. causes genital ulcerations

2. A bacterial infection that spreads venereal disease, causing pelvic inflammatory disease in women is
   a. syphilis
   b. gonorrhea
   c. cytomegalovirus
   d. herpes genitalis

3. Enlargement of the prostate gland related to hormone disturbances and age is
   a. benign hyperplasia
   b. glandular carcinoma
   c. caused by an undescended testis
   d. a malignancy

4. Benign hyperplastic prostate disease causes a(n)
   a. elevated bladder with a smooth contour
   b. irregular bladder floor contour
   c. urethral stricture resulting from gonorrhea
   d. invasion of the bladder wall

5. The screening technique used to determine cryptorchidism is
   a. nuclear medicine
   b. MRI
   c. ultrasound
   d. CT

6. An absent or ectopic testis has to be ruled out in cases of
   a. testicular torsion
   b. epididymitis
   c. syphilis
   d. cryptorchidism

7. Compromise of circulation and sudden onset of severe scrotal pain are suggestive of
   a. cryptorchidism
   b. epididymitis
   c. testicular torsion
   d. gonorrhea

8. Intratesticular arterial pulsations on a sonogram demonstrate good flow, which rules out
   a. epididymitis
   b. testicular torsion
   c. undescended testes
   d. benign prostatic hyperplasia

9. Epididymitis causes _____ on radionuclide studies.
   a. no findings
   b. a cold nodule
   c. a decreased uptake
   d. an increased uptake

10. The tumor that arises from a primitive germ cell or containing a variety of tissue is a
    a. seminoma
    b. benign hyperplasia
    c. teratoma
    d. bacterial infection

11. Normal testicular tissue is homogeneous; in cases of a seminoma, the ultrasound scan appears as
    a. an inhomogeneous cystic and solid mass with calcification
    b. increased echogenicity with uniform echoes
    c. decreased echogenicity with uniform echoes
    d. a uniform hypoechoic mass without calcification

12. Metastasis from testicular tumors typically occurs
    a. at the renal hilum
    b. where the gonadal veins drain
    c. are best detected by computed tomography
    d. all of the above

13. Venereal diseases, unsterile delivery or abortion, or complications of intrauterine devices can result in
    a. polycystic ovarian syndrome
    b. dermoid cysts
    c. pelvic inflammatory disease
    d. trophoblastic disease

14. To best demonstrate pelvic abscesses, which may cause pelvic inflammatory disease, the modality of choice is
    a. CT
    b. MRI
    c. ultrasound
    d. nuclear medicine

15. Ovarian cysts appear as
    a. calcium carbonate deposits on a plain abdominal x-ray
    b. rounded anechoic adnexal masses
    c. solid irregular areas with amorphous shadows
    d. a mass with associated ascites

16. Cystic masses with several thin, well-defined septations is suggestive of a(n)
    a. cystadenoma
    b. cystadenocarcinoma
    c. ovarian cyst
    d. metastatic ovarian tumor

17. A germ cell tumor containing hair, skin, teeth, and fatty elements is
    a. a dermoid cyst
    b. an ovarian cyst
    c. polycystic ovarian disease
    d. a seminoma

18. Dermoid cysts can be demonstrated on
    a. ultrasound as an anechoic mass
    b. ultrasound as a hypoechoic mass
    c. x-ray as a radiolucency with calcifications
    d. x-ray as a thickened bladder wall

19. A benign smooth-muscle tumor of the uterus is a
    a. fibroid
    b. cystadenoma
    c. teratoma
    d. dermoid cyst

20. The most common calcified lesion in the female genital tract is a
    a. teratoma
    b. primary cystadenocarcinoma
    c. fibroid
    d. cystadenoma

21. The invasive endometrial neoplasm of the uterine body is
    a. endometriosis
    b. endometrial carcinoma
    c. fibroids
    d. a seminoma

22. When the normal endometrium extends or appears outside the uterus it is called
    a. a teratoma
    b. fibroids
    c. endometriosis
    d. pelvic inflammatory disease

23. Poor hygiene, chronic irritation, and infection appear to be related to the development of
    a. endometriosis
    b. seminomas
    c. cervical cancer
    d. ovarian cancer

24. Diffuse enlargement of the uterine body with omental metastases is indicative of
    a. leiomyomas
    b. teratomas
    c. carcinoma of the cervix
    d. endometrial carcinoma

25. In mammography, benign breast disease appears as a
    a. mass with irregular margins
    b. smooth well-circumscribed mass without extensions
    c. mass with spiculations and calcifications
    d. snowstorm due to calcifications

26. MRI is used for patients with breast implants; breast carcinoma appears as a(n)
    a. hypoechoic lesion
    b. low signal intensity without spiculations
    c. high signal intensity with spiculations
    d. anechoic lesion within a thin echogenic capsule

27. In pregnancy, excessive amniotic fluid is seen in cases of
    a. oligohydramnios
    b. polyhydramnios
    c. hydramnios
    d. trophoblastic disease

28. In about half the patients with pelvic inflammatory disease, implantation of a fertilized ovum occurs in the
    a. fallopian tubes
    b. uterus
    c. vaginal canal
    d. omentum

29. The lack of a female chromosome causing an abnormal fertilization is known as a(n)
    a. choriocarcinoma
    b. hydatidiform mole
    c. seminoma
    d. ectopic pregnancy

30. This tumor is a trophoblastic disease, which usually appears as a large complex mass of central hemorrhage in the expected position of the uterus, is called a
    a. choriocarcinoma
    b. uterine carcinoma
    c. teratoma
    d. hydatidiform mole

12 Miscellaneous Diseases

OBJECTIVES

In addition to the objectives listed at the beginning of Chapter 12 in the textbook, the user should be able to:

1. Differentiate the pathologic disorders from the nutritional disorders and vitamin deficiencies by defining the disease processes and their radiographic manifestations.
2. Determine changes in technical factors to obtain optimal-quality radiographs for patients with various underlying pathologic conditions.
3. Describe the pathologic conditions associated with sarcoidosis, muscular dystrophy, melanoma, and systemic lupus erythematosus.
4. Differentiate hereditary abnormalities, including chromosomal aberrations and genetic amino acid disorders.
5. Locate placement for an endotracheal tube, central venous catheter, Swan-Ganz catheter, and transvenous cardiac pacemaker.
6. Recognize the most common complications involved with improper placement of the aforementioned catheters and how chest radiography plays an important role in the diagnosis of these complications.

EXERCISE 1—FILL IN THE BLANK: MISCELLANEOUS PATHOLOGY

Complete the following questions regarding nutritional diseases by writing the correct term(s) in the blank(s) provided.

1. Peripheral vasodilation causes increased _____ _____, producing generalized enlargement of the cardiac silhouette.

2. The body requires _____ to complete the cellular process called respiration.

3. Weakening of capillary walls often results in bleeding into the skin, joints, and internal organs in cases of

   _____.

4. To maintain the integrity of the mucous membrane lining the respiratory, gastrointestinal, and urogenital tracts, the

   body requires vitamin _____.

5. Calcium deposited in the kidney, heart, lungs, and stomach wall may be caused by _____.

6. Excessive eating combined with a lack of activity can result in _____.

EXERCISE 2—FILL IN THE BLANK: MISCELLANEOUS PATHOLOGY

Complete the following questions associated with the miscellaneous and hereditary diseases by writing the correct term(s) in the blank(s) provided.

1. The chronic form of _____ _____ may cause mental retardation, seizures, or delayed development.

2. Bilateral, symmetric hilar lymph node enlargement is the classic radiographic abnormality in

   _____.

3. The most frequent complaint of patients with _____ _____

   _____ is pain in multiple muscles and joints.

4. Metastatic _____ also produces multiple nodules in the lung and destructive bone lesions.

5. Muscle bundles that appear as finely striated or striped are suggestive of _____

   _____.

6. The most common trisomy disorder of all chromosomal aberrations is _____

   _____.

7. A shortened fourth metacarpal (possibly the fifth metacarpal) is a skeletal abnormality in patients afflicted with

   _____ _____.

8. An elongation and thinning of the tubular bones, most prominent in the hands and feet, may be seen in patients

   with _____ _____.

9. For the body to continue in a normal growth pattern and physiologic function, enzymes are required to control

   _____ _____ metabolism.

10. _____ causes brain atrophy as a result of the impaired conversion of phenylalanine to
    tyrosine.

11. Dense laminated calcification in multiple intervertebral disks beginning in the lumbar region is a radiographic

    appearance seen in patients with _____.

12. Renal, urethral, and bladder stones form as a result of excessive urinary excretion of several amino acids in cases

    of _____.

Match each of the following terms with the correct definition by placing the letter of the best answer in the space provided. Each question has only one correct answer. Please note that there are more terms than definitions.

1. _____ ascorbic acid deficiency

2. _____ decreased absorption of calcium

3. _____ deficiency of vitamin B_1

4. _____ essential for blood-clotting mechanism to function

5. _____ excessive adipose tissue due to more intake of calories than the body requires

6. _____ excessive intake of vitamin A characterized by multiple symptoms

7. _____ inability of gastrointestinal tract to digest and use proteins, carbohydrates, and lipids is one cause

8. _____ niacin deficiency

9. _____ produces abnormalities involving the gastrointestinal tract and nervous system

10. _____ results in night blindness

A. beriberi

B. hypervitaminosis

C. nutritional deficiency

D. obesity

E. pellagra

F. protein-calorie malnutrition

G. rickets

H. scurvy

I. vitamin A deficiency

J. vitamin D

K. vitamin K

L. vitamin K deficiency

Match each of the following terms with the correct definition by placing the letter of the best answer in the space provided. Each question has only one correct answer. Please note that there are more terms than definitions.

1. _____ complex lipids accumulate in excessive amounts in the spleen, liver, and bone marrow

2. _____ concentration deposited in the rapidly growing portions of bones, especially the metaphysis

3. _____ connective tissue disorder affecting vision, skeletal, and cardiovascular systems

4. _____ connective tissue disorder most likely representing an immune-complex disorder

5. _____ enzyme deficiency leading to an abnormal accumulation of homogentisic acid

6. _____ error of impairment to convert phenylalanine to tyrosine

7. _____ excessive urinary excretion of several amino acids

8. _____ gonadal dysgenesis, characterized by primary amenorrhea

9. _____ group of chronic inherited conditions in which fat replaces muscle

10. _____ inborn error of the metabolism of the amino acid methionine

11. _____ malignant skin cancer

12. _____ multisystem granulomatous disease

13. _____ mutation of the genes causing a disease process

14. _____ testicular dysgenesis, failure to produce sperm and testosterone

15. _____ three strands of chromosome 21 (trisomy)

A. alkaptonuria

B. arachnodactyly

C. chromosomal aberration

D. cystinuria

E. Down syndrome

F. Gaucher's disease

G. homocystinuria

H. Klinefelter's syndrome

I. kwashiorkor

J. lead poisoning

K. Marfan syndrome

L. melanoma

M. muscular dystrophy

N. Pelken's spur

O. phenylketonuria

P. sarcoidosis

Q. systemic lupus erythematosus

R. Turner's syndrome

Circle the best answer for the following multiple choice questions.

1. Beriberi is caused by a deficiency of _____, resulting in a lack of growth and muscle tone.
   a. thiamine
   b. niacin
   c. vitamin C
   d. retinol

2. The fat-soluble vitamin that is necessary to maintain the blood-clotting mechanism is
   a. vitamin D
   b. vitamin A
   c. vitamin K
   d. vitamin B_1

3. Diffuse edema, ascites, and a protuberant abdomen are clinical findings in patients with
   a. hypervitaminosis
   b. protein-calorie malnutrition
   c. obesity
   d. scurvy

4. Bilateral symmetric hilar lymph node enlargement is the classic radiographic appearance of
   a. systemic lupus erythematosus
   b. lead poisoning
   c. melanoma
   d. sarcoidosis

5. Metastases from this malignant neoplasm frequently involve the gastrointestinal tract as well-circumscribed, round, or oval nodules that may develop central necrosis and ulceration. This malignancy is
   a. sarcoidoma
   b. melanoma
   c. lupus
   d. kwashiorkor

6. Three strands of chromosome number 21 instead of the normal two result in
   a. Turner' syndrome
   b. Marfan syndrome
   c. Klinefelter's syndrome
   d. Down syndrome

7. Testicular dysgenesis is a chromosomal aberration caused by
   a. three strands of chromosome 21
   b. an inherited generalized chromosomal disorder of connective tissue
   c. one X chromosome
   d. two or more X chromosomes

8. An error in metabolism due to a genetic amino acid disorder, causing a defect in the structure of collagen or elastin, is
   a. homocystinuria
   b. phenylketonuria
   c. alkaptonuria
   d. cystinuria

9. Placement of the endotracheal tube should be evident on an x-ray at
   a. the carina
   b. 5 to 7 cm above the carina
   c. 10 to 15 cm above the carina
   d. the mainstem bronchi

10. The central venous pressure (CVP) line placement image must include
    a. the tip of the catheter on an overexposed image
    b. the tip of the catheter and the lung tissue without overexposure
    c. the tip without obscuring a possible pleural effusion or pneumothorax
    d. b and c

EXERCISE 5—CASE STUDIES

The following case studies required imaging related to the internal device placement. After each scenario, the images are presented and you will be asked to answer questions. Using the knowledge of imaging pathology and internal devices, apply exposure factors and positioning criteria to answer the questions posed.

A 45-year-old male has a clinical follow-up image in the intensive care unit, which included a portable chest x-ray, to evaluate his tracheostomy tube placement. See the portable chest image below.

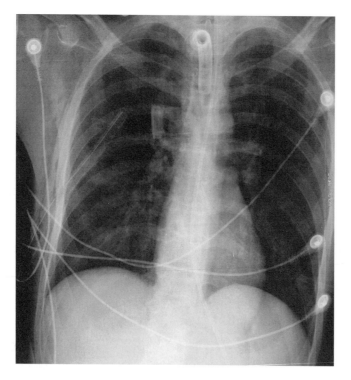

1. The purpose of the image is to locate the tracheostomy tube. Where is the tip of the tracheostomy tube?

2. The chest x-ray was taken with the patient in the recumbent position. Is this a concern when evaluating tube placement?

3. By completing the x-ray in the recumbent position, what pathology could be missed?

4. In the mobile setting, if air-fluid levels need to be demonstrated, what positioning criteria are needed?

5. What is the other tube in the right lung called?

6. What is this tube for?

CASE STUDY 2

A 40-year-old female has a clinical follow-up image in the intensive care unit, which included a portable chest x-ray, to evaluate the Swan-Ganz catheter and the tracheostomy tube placement. See the portable chest image below.

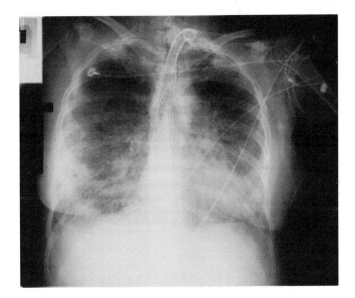

1. In this case, the external portion of the Swan-Ganz catheter is seen on the left shoulder. Can you identify the distal or internal placement of this catheter?

2. How would a radiographer determine if the proper exposure factors have been used by viewing the radiograph?

173

3. One purpose of the image is to locate the tracheostomy tube. Where is the tip of the tube demonstrated?

4. Looking closely, there is a tube that is in the patient midline from the superior (neck) chest through to the inferior chest (below the diaphragm). Because this tube appears to continue into the abdominal structures, what might this tube be?

Could this tube be the oxygen tubing?

5. What are the three lines called that are crossing off to the left of the patient?

Have these lines been moved sufficiently? Can you disconnect these lines?

A 55-year-old male was experiencing shortness of breath (SOB), so he has a clinical follow-up image. The patient previously has had a coronary artery bypass graft (CABG). The following chest image was done upright on inspiration.

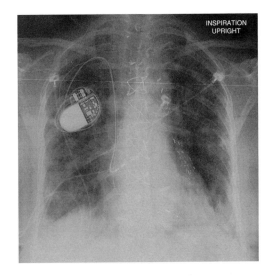

1. In viewing this image, the pulse generator (pacemaker) is seen in the right lung/shoulder region. Can you identify the distal or internal placement of the leads?

2. Are the electrocardiogram (EKG) leads interfering with identification of the pacer leads?

3. The most superior pacemaker lead would be located where?

4. The inferior pacemaker lead is located where?

Read each question carefully, then circle the best answer.

1. A deficiency in _____ will cause vision problems due to the lack of pigment in the rods of the retina.
   a. thiamine
   b. niacin
   c. vitamin D
   d. retinol

2. This water-soluble vitamin helps to produce and maintain vascular endothelium; it is
   a. vitamin B_1
   b. vitamin B_3
   c. vitamin C
   d. vitamin D

3. In hypervitaminosis, too much calcium is absorbed from the gastrointestinal tract because of excessive
   a. vitamin B_3
   b. vitamin C
   c. vitamin D
   d. vitamin K

4. Ingestion of this substance is interchangeable with calcium in the body, causing dense transverse bands in the metaphysis; it is
   a. hypervitaminosis
   b. lead
   c. vitamin K
   d. increased caloric intake

5. A connective tissue disorder having a characteristic butterfly-shaped rash over the nose is
   a. sarcoidosis
   b. melanoma
   c. hypervitaminosis
   d. systemic lupus erythematous

6. Fat that replaces muscle leads to generalized weakness and eventually causes respiratory muscle failure in
   a. muscular dystrophy
   b. multiple sclerosis
   c. sarcoidosis
   d. lupus

7. Primary amenorrhea, a result of a chromosomal aberration, is
   a. Down syndrome
   b. Turner's syndrome
   c. Marfan syndrome
   d. Klinefelter's syndrome

8. Profound retardation due to the lack of enzyme conversion to create tyrosine occurs in infants with
   a. homocystinuria
   b. cystinuria
   c. ochronosis
   d. phenylketonuria

9. Excessive quantities of complex lipids in the reticuloendothelial cells of the spleen, liver, and bone marrow is called a
   a. genetic amino acid disorder
   b. type of muscular dystrophy
   c. glycogen storage disease
   d. none of the above

10. A device that can measure the pulmonary capillary wedge pressure, cardiac output, and central venous pressure is a
    a. Swan-Ganz catheter
    b. CVP catheter
    c. peripherally inserted central catheter (PICC) line
    d. transvenous cardiac pacer

177

Answer Key

CHAPTER 1

Exercise 1—Fill in the Blank

1. pathology
2. signs
3. symptoms
4. neoplasia
5. iatrogenic
6. idiopathic
7. nosocomial
8. community acquired
9. inflammation
10. a. Alterations in blood flow and vascular permeability
    b. Migration of circulating white blood cells to the interstitium of the injured tissue
    c. Phagocytosis and enzymatic digestion of dead cells and tissue elements
    d. Repair of injury by regeneration of normal parenchymal cells or proliferation of granulation tissue and eventual scar formation
11. permeable
12. exudate
13. granulation
14. fibrous adhesion
15. keloid
16. a. rubor
    b. calor
    c. tumor
    d. dolor
    e. loss of function
17. heat (calor), redness (rubor)
18. tumor
19. pain (dolor), loss of function
20. pyogenic
21. suppurative
22. abscess
23. bacteremia
24. edema
25. anasarca
26. effusion
27. ascites
28. ischemia
29. infarct
30. infarctions
31. hemorrhage
32. hematoma
33. atrophy
34. hypoplasia, aplasia
35. disuse
36. irreversible or pathologic
37. hyperplasia
38. dysplasia
39. neoplasia
40. oncology
41. benign
42. malignant
43. cancers
44. parenchyma, stroma
45. parenchymal
46. fibroma
47. adenomas
48. carcinomas
49. glandular
50. sarcoma
51. seeding, lymphatic, hematogenic
52. seeding
53. Grading, staging
54. hereditary
55. Dominant, recessive
56. mutations
57. Antibodies
58. immunity
59. Vaccines; toxoid
60. acquired immunodeficiency syndrome (AIDS), human immunodeficiency virus (HIV)
61. hepatitis
62. B

Exercise 2—Matching

1. M	11. H
2. W	12. U
3. O	13. S
4. A	14. V
5. K	15. P
6. T	16. G
7. E	17. C
8. J	18. R
9. D	19. I
10. Q	20. B

Exercise 3—Multiple Choice

1. c	9. b
2. b	10. c
3. c	11. b
4. b	12. a
5. a	13. c
6. d	14. c
7. a	15. b
8. d	

Self-Test

1. a	7. a
2. b	8. c
3. b	9. c
4. d	10. d
5. a	11. a
6. b	12. c

179

13. b   20. a
14. c   21. d
15. d   22. a
16. d   23. b
17. d   24. d
18. b   25. b
19. b

CHAPTER 2

Exercise 1—Fill in the Blank

1. ultrasound (US)
2. ultrasound
3. computed axial tomography; computed tomography
4. computed tomography
5. magnetic resonance imaging
6. PET—positron emission tomography
7. fused or integrated
8. ultrasound
9. echoes
10. anechoic
11. hyperechoic or echogenic
12. isoechoic
13. patency of major blood vessels
14. direction, velocity
15. air; bone or barium
16. computed tomography
17. CT number
18. bone; 1000
19. lowest; air
20. 2.0 mm
21. spiral; helical
22. multidetectors
23. volume-rendered
24. echo; repetition
25. spin-echo
26. T1-weighted
27. signal void
28. intravenous contrast or gadolinium chelates
29. diffusion
30. fat-suppressed
31. nuclear medicine
32. radiopharmaceutical
33. gamma
34. hot spot
35. single-photon emission computed tomography
36. heart; strokes
37. radiopharmaceutical; positron
38. annihilation
39. oncology, cardiology
40. integrated, direct

Exercise 2—Matching

1. U   7. B
2. I   8. E
3. L   9. R
4. Q   10. C
5. Y   11. S
6. Z   12. T

13. P   17. X
14. H   18. J
15. W   19. F
16. M   20. D

Exercise 3—Multiple Choice

1. c   11. d
2. d   12. a
3. a   13. c
4. d   14. b
5. a   15. d
6. a   16. b
7. b   17. b
8. c   18. d
9. a   19. d
10. a   20. a

Self-Test

1. d   11. e
2. a   12. d
3. c   13. a
4. b   14. a
5. c   15. b
6. a   16. b
7. b   17. b
8. d   18. a
9. b   19. d
10. c   20. b

CHAPTER 3

Exercise 1—Labeling

A. Structure of the respiratory system.
1. nasal cavity
2. pharynx
3. larynx
4. trachea
5. alveoli
6. capillary
7. alveolar sac
8. alveolar duct
9. bronchioles
10. lower respiratory system
11. left and right primary bronchi
12. upper respiratory system

B. The lungs and pleura.
1. left lung
2. esophagus
3. visceral pleura
4. intrapleural space
5. pulmonary trunk
6. heart
7. sternum
8. primary bronchus
9. pulmonary vessels
10. parietal pleura
11. right lung

Exercise 2—Fill in the Blank

1. a. oxygenate blood
   b. removal of body waste
2. a. trachea
   b. bronchi
   c. bronchioles
3. conduction of air
4. mucous membrane
5. hairlike
6. Cilia
7. proliferate
8. lung parenchyma (alveoli)
9. hemoglobin; internal
10. diaphragm; intercostal; fill with air
11. body
12. visceral pleura

Exercise 3—Fill in the Blank

1. cystic fibrosis
2. Surfactant
3. Soft tissue
4. Pneumonia
5. spherical; hazy poorly defined
6. *Mycobacterium tuberculosis*
7. coccidioidomycosis
8. nosocomial
9. COPD or chronic pulmonary obstructive disease
10. silicosis
11. Bronchial adenoma
12. arteriovenous fistula

Exercise 4—Matching

1. F	7. L
2. I	8. G
3. A	9. H
4. P	10. C
5. K	11. B
6. M	12. D

Exercise 5—Matching

1. P	11. D
2. L	12. J
3. Q	13. F
4. C	14. K
5. O	15. G
6. N	16. A
7. R	17. U
8. I	18. H
9. T	19. S
10. M	20. B

Exercise 6—Multiple Choice

1. a	6. d
2. b	7. a
3. b	8. b
4. c	9. b
5. b	10. a

Exercise 7—Case Studies

Case Study 1

1. Yes
2. Gastric bubble demonstrates an air-fluid level; to get this, a horizontal x-ray beam is required
3. Increased attenuation in the right upper lobe
4. No, consolidated material, radiopaque
5. Yes, normal lung tissue is well demonstrated as well as the affected area
6. Lobar pneumonia was the radiologist's differential diagnosis

Case Study 2

1. Yes, a consolidated left lung with a mediastinal shift to the right
2. No rotation, symmetrical sternoclavicular joints assuring that mediastinal shift is due to pathology not positioning error
3. Air-fluid level in the stomach
4. Decubitus with a horizontal beam; affected or fluid side down, left lateral decubitus in this case; both decubitus projections might be of benefit so may be requested
5. Coccidioidomycosis (fungal)—pulmonary mycosis

Self-Test

1. b		16. a
2. b		17. b
3. d		18. d
4. d		19. b
5. a		20. d
6. c		21. a
7. b		22. c
8. a		23. c
9. c		24. a
10. b		25. a
11. c		26. a
12. a		27. c
13. a		28. d
14. b		29. a
15. a		30. c

CHAPTER 4

Exercise 1—Labeling

A. Long bone.
   1. articular cartilage
   2. spongy bone
   3. epiphyseal plate
   4. red marrow cavities
   5. compact bone
   6. medullary cavity
   7. endosteum
   8. yellow marrow
   9. periosteum
   10. epiphysis
   11. diaphysis
   12. epiphysis

B. Bone fracture and repair.
1. fracture
2. bleeding
3. bony callus
4. repaired bone

Exercise 2—Fill in the Blank

1. a. bone
   b. cartilage
2. a. compact bone (dense or cortical bone)
   b. cancellous bone (spongy bone)
3. a. outer covering—periosteum
   b. inner lining—endosteum
4. dense; structureless
5. cancellous; spongy
6. trabeculae
7. epiphyseal
8. osteoblasts; osteoclasts
9. ossification; resorption
10. intramembranous ossification
11. osteoblasts
12. a. supporting frame
    b. protects vital organs
    c. levers for movement
    d. produce blood cells in the red marrow
    e. storage of calcium

Exercise 3—Fill in the Blank

1. transitional
2. spina bifida
3. achondroplasia
4. Osteoarthritis
5. Bursitis
6. osteomyelitis
7. mineralization
8. Paget's
9. aneurysmal
10. callus
11. malunion
12. Rheumatoid arthritis

Exercise 4—Matching

1. J		7. A	
2. G		8. D	
3. B		9. H	
4. I		10. L	
5. F		11. C	
6. M		12. O	

Exercise 5—Matching

1. Q		9. T	
2. W		10. L	
3. F		11. I	
4. C		12. A	
5. P		13. N	
6. D		14. B	
7. J		15. U	
8. K		16. O	

17. R	19. G
18. E	20. X

Exercise 6—Matching

1. F		7. A	
2. C		8. G	
3. D		9. N	
4. K		10. B	
5. M		11. J	
6. I		12. E	

Exercise 7—Matching

1. I		6. G	
2. F		7. J	
3. B		8. A	
4. D		9. H	
5. E		10. C	

Exercise 8—Multiple Choice

1. b		7. b	
2. a		8. a	
3. b		9. a	
4. c		10. b	
5. d		11. b	
6. d		12. d	

Exercise 9—Case Studies

Case Study 1

1. A. CR enters the head of the third metacarpal
   B. The hand is placed with the palmar surface on the image receptor so the coronal plane is parallel to the image receptor
2. Any of the following four suggestions might be alternatives to improve the image.
   A. Ball catcher's projection
   B. AP
   C. Do each hand separately
   D. Do not force the patient because it may result in a fracture
3. An inflammatory process
4. Differential diagnosis; psoriatic arthritis

Case Study 2

1. The epiphyseal growth plate proximally and distally is evidence the person is still growing.
2. Slight superimposition of the tibia and fibula both proximally and distally would indicate a true AP was completed.
No, the leg is not in a true AP.
The proximal and distal tibia and fibula are too superimposed, indicating lateral rotation.
3. A radiolucency is visualized on the proximal fibula.
4. By adding the second perspective, the radiolucency (size and location) is more readily visualized.
5. Yes
No, the images demonstrate soft tissue, bony trabeculae, and cortical bone.

6. The lucency would be caused by some sort of bone erosion.
7. Differential diagnosis—bone cyst: aneurysmal or unicameral

Case Study 3

1. The following is visualized on the dorsoplantar projection:
    A. Artifact on the proximal shaft of the fifth metatarsal
    B. Tarsals are demonstrated with good bony trabeculae visible, indicating that the technique was adjusted to demonstrate this area of interest
    C. Toes are difficult to visualize—overexposed
2. No, overexposed—for better visibility of detail, one of the following would be recommended
    A. Add a filter to attenuate a portion of the x-ray beam at the toes
    B. Increase the kV and lower the mAs to produce the same density and decrease the contrast
3. On the oblique, there is a fracture of the base on the fifth metatarsal—Jones fracture
4. The base of the fifth metatarsal is well visualized, providing a second perspective of the fracture; however the foot is rotated. To correct this error adjust the plantar surface perpendicular to the image receptor.
5. It may require 2 to 3 perspectives to demonstrate all anatomic structures without superimposition.
6. Differential diagnosis—Jones fracture

Case Study 4

1. The vertebral bodies; anterior and posterior arches of C1 are displaced.
2. Jefferson fracture, which is a comminuted fracture of the ring of the atlas involving the anterior and posterior arches with displacement.
3. If axial projections are a requirement of the protocol requested, the technologist only changed the sequence of completing the series—this is usually an acceptable practice.
4. No, because the radiographer is uncomfortable with placing the patient in hyperextension does not permit a change in orders without a physician's order—this is outside their scope of practice. Two alternatives:
    A. The radiographer can speak with the radiologist and discuss the alternatives; in some cases the axial projections may be ordered.
    B. The resident could be asked to hyperextend the patient, with monitoring for neurologic deficits; if they occur the procedure could be stopped.
** In this case it was fortunate for all parties involved that the axial images were completed first and evaluated to prevent any permanent neurologic damage.

Self-Test

1. b or d depending upon protocol	12. a
2. d	13. b
3. a	14. d
4. b	15. a
5. a	16. a
6. d	17. b
7. a	18. a
8. a	19. d
9. c	20. d
10. b	21. a
11. b	22. a

CHAPTER 5

Exercise 1—Labeling

A. Location of the digestive organs.
    1. tongue
    2. larynx
    3. trachea
    4. cystic duct
    5. hepatic duct
    6. spleen
    7. pancreas
    8. duodenum
    9. gallbladder
    10. liver
    11. stomach
    12. left colic flexure
    13. descending colon
    14. sigmoid colon
    15. anal canal
    16. rectum
    17. vermiform appendix
    18. cecum
    19. iliem
    20. ascending colon
    21. right colic flexure
    22. transverse colon
    23. diaphragm
    24. esophagus
    25. pharynx
    26. salivary glands
B. Stomach.
    1. fundus
    2. body of stomach
    3. serosa
    4. muscularis
    5. gastric mucosa
    6. greater curvature
    7. rugae or gastric folds
    8. duodenum
    9. duodenal bulb
    10. pyloric sphincter
    11. pylorus

183

12. lesser curvature
13. lower esophageal sphincter
14. gastroesophageal opening
15. esophagus
C. Divisions of the large intestine.
    1. transverse colon
    2. left colic flexure
    3. descending colon
    4. sigmoid colon
    5. anus
    6. external anal sphincter muscle
    7. rectum
    8. ileum
    9. vermiform appendix
    10. cecum
    11. ileocecal valve
    12. ascending colon
    13. right colic flexure
    14. superior mesenteric artery
D. Ducts that carry bile from the liver and gallbladder.
    1. common hepatic duct
    2. common bile duct
    3. pancreas
    4. pancreatic duct
    5. hepatopancreatic sphincter
    6. duodenum
    7. duodenal papilla
    8. cystic duct
    9. liver
    10. neck of gallbladder
    11. corpus (body) of gallbladder

Exercise 2—Fill in the Blank

1. chemical; physical
2. absorbed; used
3. a. endocrine
   b. exocrine
4. mouth; mastication
5. deglutition
6. chyme
7. peristalsis
8. emulsification
9. protein
10. intestinal wall
11. a. vitamin A
    b. vitamin D
    c. vitamin E
    d. vitamin K
12. insulin; glucagon

Exercise 3—Fill in the Blank

1. tracheoesophageal fistula
2. gastroesophageal reflux
3. corrosive agents
4. Zenker's
5. varices
6. perforation
7. gastritis
8. pepsin; peptic ulcer or ulcer
9. Crohn's

10. mechanical
11. adynamic ileus
12. appendicitis
13. carcinoma
14. ulcerative colitis
15. colon cancer
16. acute cholecystitis
17. porcelain; carcinoma
18. CT
19. pathognomonic
20. perforation; ulcer

Exercise 4—Matching

1.	F	7.	B
2.	J	8.	I
3.	A	9.	K
4.	H	10.	M
5.	N	11.	G
6.	L	12.	D

Exercise 5—Matching

1.	K	9.	N
2.	O	10.	F
3.	H	11.	P
4.	J	12.	G
5.	Q	13.	L
6.	M	14.	C
7.	A	15.	E
8.	B	16.	D

Exercise 6—Matching

1.	D	7.	F
2.	N	8.	O
3.	E	9.	H
4.	A	10.	B
5.	I	11.	J
6.	G	12.	P

Exercise 7—Matching

1.	C	6.	G
2.	E	7.	J
3.	K	8.	I
4.	F	9.	B
5.	L	10.	A

Exercise 8—Multiple Choice

1.	b	11.	b
2.	a	12.	a
3.	a	13.	b
4.	d	14.	d
5.	d	15.	b
6.	a	16.	a
7.	c	17.	a
8.	c	18.	d
9.	d	19.	b
10.	a	20.	a

Exercise 9—Case Studies

Case Study 1

1. Usually only one parent is allowed to assist as both do not need to receive radiation exposure. However, if department protocol or radiologist preference is to have the parents not assist, then the radiographer needs to communicate this to the parents in a politically correct manner. In some cases, parents are more of a hindrance than help in getting a procedure completed.
2. The use of sterile water to dilute the barium is suggested to minimize possible infection. The amount of water required will depend on the W/V concentration the radiologist requests. In infants, the concentration of barium is slightly lower than for adults.
3. A nasogastric or feeding tube has been gently placed in the pharynx so as not to cause a perforation and to visualize anatomic structures.
4. Oropharynx and laryngopharynx, which demonstrates a blunt pouch (proximal esophagus)
5. Esophageal atresia or transesophageal fistula

Case Study 2

1. Inflammation and fibrosis cause rigid thickening of the bowel wall, resulting in a narrowing
2. The "string sign" is seen in multiple areas of the small bowel
3. Skip lesions
4. Crohn's disease
5. The radiologist is trying to move the barium through the small bowel and demonstrate the diseased portion of the small bowel.
6. The formation of fistulas

Case Study 3

1. Intussusception
2. The coiled spring is a result of the bowel telescoping within itself (like a slinky).
3. The contrast/barium has moved slightly further into the colon. In this case, the radiologist externally manipulated the bowel.
4. a. The enema bag should run by gravity flow being approximately 24 inches above the table.
   b. To assure that perforation will not occur due to increased pressure as a result of the enema.
5. The intussusception has been relieved; the bowel is now fully filled.
6. Both—diagnostic in demonstrating the pathologic condition and therapeutic in relieving the telescoping bowel.
   The infant was relieved of the intussusception upon completion of the barium enema; however, the bowel relapsed the following day and surgery had to be performed.

Case Study 4

1. Air-fluid level in the stomach
2. It is recommended that the patient be in the upright position for a minimum of 5 minutes (10 to 20 minutes is preferred) to form air-fluid levels.
3. Place the patient into the required position before completing any other procedural criteria. When completing the remaining steps, the expected time frame will pass so the image will demonstrate air-fluid levels.
4. Any and all upright images should be completed first to ensure air-fluid levels. In this case, the patient already has air-fluid levels from sitting; doing the upright imaging first is more efficient in this case.
5. Yes, under both diaphragms. There is air pushing down the stomach and liver.
6. Pneumoperitoneum
7. A left lateral decubitus

Self-Test

1. c		14. a
2. a		15. b
3. b		16. d
4. d		17. b
5. a		18. c
6. c		19. a
7. c		20. c
8. d		21. a
9. a		22. b
10. d		23. b
11. b		24. a
12. c		25. c
13. b		

CHAPTER 6

Exercise 1—Labeling

A. Location of the urinary system.
   1. renal artery
   2. renal vein
   3. left kidney
   4. abdominal aorta
   5. inferior vena cava
   6. urethra
   7. urinary bladder
   8. ureter
   9. right kidney
   10. liver
   11. adrenal gland
B. Internal structure of the kidney.
   1. fibrous capsule
   2. cortex
   3. minor calyces
   4. major calyces
   5. medullary pyramid
   6. medulla
   7. ureter
   8. renal papilla of pyramid
   9. renal pelvis
   10. hilum
   11. renal sinus
C. Structure and location of the male urinary bladder.
   1. peritoneum (cut away)
   2. smooth muscle

185

3. trigone
4. ureteral opening (L)
5. internal urinary sphincter
6. urethra
7. external urinary sphincter
8. prostate gland
9. rugae
10. ureteral opening (R)

Exercise 2—Fill in the Blank

1. waste products; reabsorb; secrete
2. nephron
3. glomerulus
4. proximal convoluted tubule
5. a. descending limb
   b. loop
   c. ascending limb
6. electrolyte; acid base
7. papillae
8. renal pelvis
9. reservoir
10. right ureter; left ureter; urethra
11. trigone
12. void; micturate
13. urethra
14. ureterovesical junction
15. incontinence

Exercise 3—Fill in the Blank

1. compensatory hypertrophy
2. malrotated
3. ureterocele
4. duplication
5. horseshoe kidney
6. glomerulonephritis
7. tuberculosis
8. papillary necrosis
9. kidney stones
10. staghorn
11. hydroureter
12. a. ureteropelvic junction
    b. ureterovesical junction
    c. bladder neck
    d. urethral meatus
13. renal cyst
14. polycystic kidney
15. a. hematuria
    b. flank pain
    c. possibly palpable abdominal mass
16. renal carcinoma
17. Wilms' tumor
18. carcinoma
19. renal vein thrombosis
20. chronic renal failure

Exercise 4—Matching

1. F
2. N
3. H
4. B
5. M
6. J

7. O
8. I
9. D
10. E
11. G
12. C

Exercise 5—Matching

1. T
2. R
3. S
4. I
5. G
6. H
7. K
8. N
9. Q
10. B
11. P
12. D
13. E
14. U
15. F
16. O
17. J
18. M
19. C
20. L

Exercise 6—Multiple Choice

1. b
2. a
3. b
4. a
5. a
6. a
7. b
8. d
9. a
10. d
11. c
12. a
13. d
14. b
15. d
16. c
17. c
18. c

Exercise 7—Case Studies

Case Study 1

1. On the left, there is a radiolucent line on the posterior aspect of the contrast-enhanced kidney. Posterior to the kidney, blood representing a hematoma is seen as an area more radiolucent than the opaque contrast-enhanced kidney.
2. Yes, the blood does not enhance and the kidney does due to the vascularity of the kidney.
3. Kidney fracture with a hematoma
4. A hematoma or bleeding from the trauma
5. Right kidney—contrast-enhanced kidney parenchyma and renal pelvis are anterior to the mass. The kidney has lost the smooth contour because of the hematoma.
6. Differential diagnosis—large renal hematoma on the right positioned posterior to the kidney.

Case Study 2

1. To demonstrate the bowel preparation in scheduled cases and if any pathology is evident before the contrast injection, it will be visualized.
2. In the left kidney tissue (cortex or parenchyma), there is evidence of a renal calculus (radiopaque).
3. If there is a blockage, there will be reduced drainage causing the kidney to stay contrast-enhanced for a longer period of time. The renal calculus may be obscured by the contrast due to similar attenuation factors between the contrast and the stone.

4. There are two radiopaque objects in the area of the bladder.
5. No, the objects will be obscured by the contrast agent.
6. Differential diagnosis—stones in the bladder lodged in diverticula
Phleboliths are a possibility on initial film; must demonstrate that the stones are in the bladder

Case Study 3

1. Foley catheter is used to fill the bladder in the retrograde approach.
2. To ensure that the bladder is filling without complication
3. The bladder outline is normal for the patient's age; on the right inferior, there is an extension of the bladder that is questionable
4. Extends inferiorly through a "neck" on the right side.
5. Whether the lesion was located anteriorly or posteriorly in reference to the bladder. In this case, the filling defect is anteriorly located.
6. There is a filling defect inferior to the bladder with connection—questionable fistula or herniation.
Differential radiologic diagnosis—16.0 cm × 9.0 cm mass in the right scrotum, which is compatible with a bladder herniation or large diverticulum projecting through the inguinal canal in the right side of the scrotum.

Self-Test

1. c	11. c
2. b	12. a
3. a	13. c
4. a	14. b
5. c	15. a
6. b	16. d
7. b	17. a
8. c	18. b
9. d	19. a
10. a	20. b

CHAPTER 7

Exercise 1—Labeling

A. Conduction system of the heart and vascular anatomy.
1. aortic arch
2. pulmonary artery
3. pulmonary veins
4. mitral (bicuspid) valve
5. Purkinje fibers
6. left ventricle
7. bundle of His
8. inferior vena cava
9. right ventricle
10. tricuspid valve
11. right atrium
12. atrioventricular (AV) node
13. pulmonary veins
14. sinoatrial (SA) node
15. superior vena cava
B. Principal arteries.
1. left common carotid a.
2. left subclavian a.
3. aortic arch
4. pulmonary a.
5. left coronary a.
6. aorta
7. splenic a.
8. renal a.
9. radial a.
10. ulnar a.
11. dorsal pedis
12. dorsal metatarsal a.
13. posterior tibial a.
14. peroneal a.
15. anterior tibial a.
16. femoral a.
17. deep femoral a.
18. external iliac a.
19. internal iliac a.
20. common iliac a.
21. abdominal aorta
22. brachial a.
23. axillary a.
24. right coronary a.
25. brachiocephalic a.
26. right common carotid a.
C. Structure of the heart valves.
1. left atrioventricular valve or mitral valve (open)
2. pulmonary semilunar valve (open on B, closed on A)
3. aortic semilunar valve (open on B, closed on A)
4. left atrioventricular valve or mitral valve (closed)
5. right atrioventricular valve or tricuspid valve (open)
6. right atrioventricular valve or tricuspid valve (closed)

Exercise 2—Fill in the Blank

1. supply; blood
2. rhythmic contractions
3. autonomic
4. Epinephrine
5. a. right atria
   b. right ventricle
   c. left atria
   d. left ventricle
6. regurgitation or backflow
7. smooth muscle
8. cusps; right; right
9. ventricles; heart
10. Systemic
11. Pulmonary
12. Systemic; left
13. diastole
14. SA node; AV node

187

Exercise 3—Fill in the Blank

1. ventricular septal defect
2. Patent ductus arteriosus
3. a. high ventricular septal defect
   b. overriding of the aortic orifice; above the ventricular defect
   c. pulmonary stenosis
   d. right ventricular hypertrophy
4. Coarctation
5. fatty
6. myocardial infarction
7. left
8. dilate or open
9. a. cardiac enlargement
   b. redistribution of pulmonary venous flow
   c. interstitial and alveolar edema
   d. pleural effusion
10. a. not using a 72″ SID
    b. performing AP versus PA projections
    c. recumbent versus upright positioning
11. cardiothoracic (C/T)
12. pulmonary venous
13. pulmonary edema
14. a. cardiac output
    b. total peripheral resistance
15. a. saccular
    b. fusiform
16. calcification
17. massive hemorrhaging
18. a. right displacement of nasogastric tube
    b. widening of the right paratracheal stripe
    c. apical pleura cap sign
19. thrombus
20. Echocardiography

Exercise 4—Matching

1. A	7. F
2. D	8. P
3. J	9. O
4. N	10. M
5. I	11. K
6. C	12. L

Exercise 5—Matching

1. S	11. H
2. Q	12. K
3. C	13. U
4. V	14. I
5. O	15. G
6. W	16. D
7. B	17. J
8. R	18. A
9. F	19. E
10. L	20. P

Exercise 6—Multiple Choice

1. a	11. c
2. c	12. a
3. a	13. d
4. a	14. d
5. c	15. d
6. d	16. a
7. d	17. c
8. b	18. a
9. d	19. b
10. a	20. a

Exercise 7—Case Studies

Case Study 1

1. For this image the patient was AP erect; the labeling was provided by the technologist who produced the image.
2. The heart may appear enlarged as a result of the AP positioning; however, the image is marked as such so the radiologist can account for this change. The heart is a greater distance from the IR, creating OID = magnification.
Yes, because the image has been labeled with the difference.
3. Decreased SID—do we know what SID was used?
Recumbent versus erect—the heart will appear larger in a recumbent image.
4. Cardiomegaly; congestive heart failure
5. The size of the patient's fist on an upright image.
No, it is enlarged laterally in both directions.
6. Cardiothoracic ratio—the heart should be less than 50% of the thoracic cavity width.

Case Study 2

1. No
2. Calcium deposits, which are common in the aorta—sometimes seen in the iliac and carotid arteries.
3. Yes, calcium (bone) is radiopaque—described on a KUB as a linear calcification outlining the aortic wall.
4. Enlarged or greater than normal
5. Pelvis
6. The iliac arteries
7. Yes, on the left in the iliac artery. The aneurysm extends into the iliac arteries.

Self-Test

1. d	12. b
2. b	13. b
3. c	14. c
4. a	15. a
5. d	16. b
6. a	17. a
7. a	18. c
8. d	19. b
9. d	20. d
10. a	21. c
11. c	22. a

23. b	27. b
24. a	28. a
25. b	29. c
26. c	30. a

CHAPTER 8

Exercise 1—Labeling

A. Structure of a neuron.
1. dendrite
2. mitochondrion
3. cell body
4. nucleus
5. axon
6. myelin sheath
7. synapse

B. Coverings and structures of the central nervous system.
1. white matter
2. gray matter
3. spinal nerve
4. dura mater
5. arachnoid
6. pia mater
7. autonomic ganglion
8. spinal cord
9. dura mater
10. arachnoid
11. pia mater
12. ventral/dorsal root

C. Divisions of the brain.
1. cerebrum
2. cortex
3. corpus callosum
4. cerebellum
5. brainstem
6. medulla oblongata
7. pons
8. midbrain
9. hypothalamus
10. pineal body
11. thalamus
12. diencephalon

Exercise 2—Fill in the Blank

1. peripheral nervous system (PNS)
2. Afferent
3. central nervous system (CNS); peripheral effectors
4. autonomic
5. neuron
6. axon
7. myelin sheath
8. synapse
9. reflux arc
10. motor or efferent
11. cortex
12. cerebrum
13. gyri
14. White

15. sensory; motor
16. Visual
17. opposite
18. corpus callosum
19. basal ganglia
20. brainstem
21. cerebellum
22. cranial bones or skull
23. a. pia mater
    b. arachnoid membrane
    c. dura mater
24. aqueduct of Sylvius
25. foramen of Monro
26. lateral
27. tentorium cerebri
28. thalamus
29. a. central nervous system
    b. peripheral nervous system
30. a. third ventricle
    b. thalamus
    c. hypothalamus

Exercise 3—Fill in the Blank

1. viral meningitis
2. meningitis
3. encephalitis
4. *Haemophilus influenzae;* pneumococci; meningococci
5. brain abscess
6. MRI
7. epidural
8. a. subdural empyema
    b. epidural empyema
9. diastatic
10. depressed
11. a. subdural
    b. epidural
    c. subarachnoid
    d. intracerebral
12. biconvex
13. subdural
14. cerebral contusions
15. subarachnoid hemorrhage
16. fracture
17. blowout; CT
18. zygomatic arch
19. tripod
20. mandible
21. nasal bones
22. cerebrovascular disease
23. rule out or exclude
24. TIA or transient ischemic attacks
25. duplex color or Doppler
26. intraparenchymal

Exercise 4—Fill in the Blank

1. MRI
2. neoplasm or tumor
3. acoustic neuroma
4. chromophobe adenoma
5. Craniopharyngiomas

189

6. germinomas; teratomas
7. chordoma
8. metastatic carcinoma
9. Petit mal
10. FDG-PET
11. normal aging
12. a. stooped posture
    b. stiff and slow movement
    c. fixed facial expression
    d. involuntary rhythmic limb tremor
13. Huntington's
14. a. noncommunicating
    b. normal pressure
15. sinusitis

Exercise 5—Matching

1. H	6. G
2. F	7. D
3. I	8. K
4. E	9. C
5. L	10. J

Exercise 6—Matching

1. C	10. P
2. E	11. I
3. W	12. G
4. H	13. Z
5. D	14. M
6. Q	15. X
7. N	16. T
8. B	17. S
9. F	18. K

Exercise 7—Matching

1. I	11. Q
2. H	12. A
3. F	13. S
4. M	14. E
5. L	15. D
6. B	16. O
7. C	17. J
8. T	18. P
9. U	19. R
10. K	20. G

Exercise 8—Matching

1. O	10. L
2. F	11. J
3. G	12. H
4. S	13. B
5. I	14. Q
6. M	15. D
7. A	16. N
8. K	17. T
9. R	18. C

Exercise 9—Multiple Choice

1. a	11. a
2. d	12. a
3. b	13. c
4. c	14. b
5. d	15. c
6. a	16. a
7. c	17. d
8. b	18. d
9. a	19. a
10. c	20. b

Exercise 10—Case Studies

Case Study 1

1. Left upper hilar region
2. Conventional tomography, CT, MRI
3. a. The greater the arc (40 degrees), the thinner the slice.
   b. Exposure time must be adequate to expose the image receptor during the full arc to produce the thinnest slice.
4. Abscess; in this case the cause was tuberculosis.
5. A ring of contrast enhancement outlining the abscess capsule.

Case Study 2

1. Carotid
2. Carotid endarterectomy
3. Aneurysm

Case Study 3

1. Cerebrovascular malformation
2. The vessels that were feeding the region were occluded or blocked.

Case Study 4

1. Cerebrospinal fluid
2. Hydrocephalus; noncommunicating and normal pressure
3. Ventricular shunt to drain the CSF to the abdominal peritoneum or the cardiovascular system
4. CT for the ventricular and sulcus size and MRI for the disorder causing the obstruction

Self-Test

1. c	11. b
2. a	12. b
3. c	13. d
4. a	14. a
5. c	15. b
6. b	16. a
7. b	17. d
8. a	18. b
9. b	19. c
10. b	20. d

CHAPTER 9

Exercise 1—Labeling

1. red blood cells (erythrocytes)
2. platelets (thrombocytes)
3. white blood cells (leukocytes)
4. granular leukocytes
5. basophil
6. neutrophil
7. eosinophil
8. nongranular leukocytes
9. lymphocyte
10. monocyte

Exercise 2—Fill in the Blank

1. a. oxygen
   b. nutrients
   c. salts
   d. hormones
2. a. infection
   b. toxic substances
   c. foreign antigens
3. a. red bone marrow
   b. lymph nodes
4. a. erythrocytes (red blood cells)
   b. thrombocytes (platelets)
   c. leukocytes (white blood cells)
5. a. red bone marrow
   b. lymphoid tissue
6. a. neutrophils (55%-75%)
   b. eosinophils (1%-4%)
   c. basophil (up to 1%)
   d. lymphocyte (25%-40%)
   e. monocytes (2%-8%)
7. neutrophil
8. platelet

Exercise 3—Fill in the Blank

1. anemia
2. a. spherocytosis
   b. sickle cell anemia
   c. thalassemia
3. sickle cell
4. thalassemia
5. Megaloblastic
6. secondary polycythemia
7. myelocytic leukemia
8. lymphatic leukemia
9. leukemia
10. lymphomas
11. a. lymph nodes
    b. spleen
    c. lymphoid tissue of parenchymal organs
12. Hodgkin's disease
13. lymph nodes
14. non-Hodgkin's lymphoma
15. mediastinum
16. PET
17. mononucleosis

18. a. platelets
    b. calcium
    c. 12 co-enzymes and proteins
19. Purpura

Exercise 4—Matching

1. F	5. J
2. E	6. D
3. H	7. K
4. A	8. B

Exercise 5—Matching

1. D	7. A
2. N	8. H
3. B	9. M
4. G	10. E
5. K	11. C
6. F	12. L

Exercise 6—Multiple Choice

1. c	6. b
2. b	7. d
3. a	8. a
4. a	9. d
5. a	10. c

Exercise 7—Case Study

1. Hodgkin's usually originates in the lymph nodes, whereas in non-Hodgkin's, the parenchymal organs are involved (approximately 40% are extranodal).
2. CT—R/O retroperitoneal adenopathy in the chest, abdomen, and pelvis

   MRI & PET—demonstrate lymphomatous involvement of the abdomen and pelvic nodes

   US—abdominal retroperitoneal adenopathy

   PET—microscopic tumor foci and altered function within normal-size nodes
3. Transversely—8.9 cm; AP diameter 10.4 cm
4. Region 1 = CT number 60; Region 2 = CT number 85; Region 3 = CT number negative 101
5. Region 1
6. Region 3

Self-Test

1. b	6. c
2. b	7. a
3. c	8. a
4. d	9. b
5. a	10. a

CHAPTER 10

Exercise 1—Labeling

A. Adrenal gland.
   1. adrenal gland
   2. kidney
   3. capsule

4. cortex
5. medulla
B. Pituitary and hormones.
   1. posterior pituitary gland
   2. antidiuretic hormone (ADH)
   3. oxytocin (OT)
   4. gonadotropic hormones (FSH and LH)
   5. thyroid-stimulating hormone (TSH)
   6. adrenocorticotropic hormone (ACTH)
   7. growth hormone (GH)
   8. anterior pituitary gland
C. Thyroid and parathyroid glands.
   1. hyoid bone
   2. larynx
   3. superior parathyroid gland
   4. thyroid gland
   5. isthmus
   6. inferior parathyroid glands
   7. trachea

Exercise 2—Fill in the Blank

1. adrenal gland
2. Mineralocorticoids
3. carbohydrate metabolism
4. a. masculinize the body
   b. retain amino acids
   c. enhance protein synthesis
5. epinephrine, norepinephrine
6. hypothalamus
7. sella turcica
8. body, development
9. posterior, smooth muscle
10. thyroxine
11. thyroid gland
12. parathyroid glands
13. a. increased calcium absorption
    b. prevents loss of calcium
    c. secretes calcitonin
14. Diabetes mellitus

Exercise 3—Fill in the Blank

1. Cushing's syndrome
2. aldosteronism
3. adrenogenital
4. adrenal
5. biochemical tests
6. neuroblastomas
7. hyperpituitarism
8. gigantism
9. Hypopituitarism
10. diabetes insipidus
11. nuclear medicine
12. benign thyroid adenoma
13. a. papillary
    b. follicular
    c. medullary
14. a. primary
    b. secondary
    c. tertiary
15. Diabetes mellitus

Exercise 4—Matching

1.	P	9.	E
2.	J	10.	I
3.	M	11.	L
4.	R	12.	C
5.	A	13.	B
6.	Q	14.	D
7.	O	15.	N
8.	G		

Exercise 5—Matching

1.	I	11.	M
2.	G	12.	H
3.	E	13.	R
4.	F	14.	C
5.	J	15.	D
6.	N	16.	W
7.	O	17.	K
8.	U	18.	B
9.	V	19.	P
10.	S	20.	T

Exercise 6—Multiple Choice

1.	c	9.	b
2.	a	10.	b
3.	d	11.	a
4.	a	12.	a
5.	b	13.	b
6.	b	14.	a
7.	b	15.	c
8.	d		

Self-Test

1.	d	13.	c
2.	a	14.	c
3.	b	15.	d
4.	a	16.	c
5.	d	17.	c
6.	a	18.	a
7.	a	19.	a
8.	c	20.	a
9.	b	21.	a
10.	b	22.	b
11.	b	23.	b
12.	c	24.	a

CHAPTER 11

Exercise 1—Labeling

A. The male reproductive system.
   1. vas deferens
   2. seminal vesicle
   3. ejaculatory duct
   4. inguinal canal
   5. spermatic cord
   6. scrotum (skin)
   7. testis
   8. epididymis

9. penis
10. vas deferens
11. prostate portion of urethra
12. prostate gland
13. urinary bladder
14. ureter
B. The female reproductive system.
   1. isthmus of uterine tube
   2. ovarian ligament
   3. ampulla of uterine tube
   4. infundibulum of uterine tube
   5. fimbriae
   6. broad ligament
   7. uterine artery and vein
   8. vagina
   9. os of vaginal cervix
   10. cervix of uterus
   11. myometrium
   12. endometrium
   13. body of uterus
   14. uterine body cavity
   15. fundus of uterus
C. The female breast.
   1. clavicle
   2. pectoralis minor muscle
   3. intercostal muscle
   4. pectoralis major muscle
   5. alveolus
   6. ductule
   7. duct
   8. lactiferous duct
   9. alveoli
   10. lactiferous sinus
   11. areola
   12. nipple pores
   13. nipple
   14. adipose tissue
   15. suspensory ligaments of Cooper

Exercise 2—Fill in the Blank

1. formation; sperm
2. spermatozoa
3. anterior lobe of the pituitary gland
4. testosterone
5. epididymis
6. vas deferens
7. seminal vesicle
8. vasectomy
9. seminal vesicles
10. a. number of sperm
    b. size of sperm
    c. shape of sperm
    d. motility of sperm
11. Menarche
12. ovulation
13. progesterone
14. fallopian tubes (uterine)
15. ectopic pregnancy
16. proliferative (postmenstrual)
17. secretory (postovulation)
18. a. blood
    b. mucus
    c. sloughed endometrium
19. menopause
20. hysterectomy

Exercise 3—Fill in the Blank

1. nonitching rash
2. Gonorrhea
3. benign prostatic hyperplasia
4. MRI
5. epididymitis
6. seminoma
7. pelvic inflammatory disease
8. infertility, ectopic pregnancy
9. dermoid cyst
10. uterine fibroids
11. endometrial carcinoma
12. hormonal changes
13. Pap smear
14. breast cancer
15. fibroadenoma
16. ultrasound
17. polyhydramnios
18. fallopian tubes
19. hydatidiform
20. choriocarcinoma

Exercise 4—Matching

1. E		7. M	
2. F		8. O	
3. B		9. H	
4. D		10. J	
5. G		11. K	
6. L		12. N	

Exercise 5—Matching

1. W		13. H	
2. G		14. R	
3. Z		15. N	
4. V		16. C	
5. B		17. J	
6. F		18. K	
7. D		19. Y	
8. S		20. U	
9. T		21. E	
10. I		22. X	
11. A		23. P	
12. Q			

Exercise 6—Multiple Choice

1. a		9. b	
2. b		10. a	
3. c		11. d	
4. d		12. a	
5. b		13. d	
6. c		14. b	
7. d		15. c	
8. b			

Exercise 7—Case Study

Case Study 1

1. Kidneys, ureters, and bladder—The superior symphysis pubis should be included.
2. The selection of the proper kVp range; near 70 kVp is necessary to differentiate soft tissue structures
3. Yes, in the right pelvis inlet/outlet, there are radiolucencies appearing as teeth.
4. Dermoid cyst

Self-Test

1. b	16. a
2. b	17. a
3. a	18. c
4. a	19. a
5. c	20. c
6. d	21. b
7. c	22. c
8. b	23. c
9. d	24. c
10. c	25. b
11. d	26. c
12. d	27. b
13. c	28. a
14. c	29. b
15. b	30. a

CHAPTER 12

Exercise 1—Fill in the Blank

1. cardiac output
2. niacin (or vitamin B_3)
3. scurvy
4. A
5. hypervitaminosis
6. obesity

Exercise 2—Fill in the Blank

1. lead poisoning
2. sarcoidosis
3. systemic lupus erythematosus
4. melanoma
5. muscular dystrophy
6. Down syndrome
7. Turner's syndrome
8. Marfan's syndrome
9. amino acid
10. Phenylketonuria
11. alkaptonuria
12. cystinuria

Exercise 3—Matching

1. H	6. B
2. G	7. C
3. A	8. E
4. K	9. F
5. D	10. I

Exercise 4—Matching

1. F	9. M
2. J	10. G
3. K	11. L
4. Q	12. P
5. A	13. C
6. O	14. H
7. D	15. E
8. R	

Exercise 5—Multiple Choice

1. a	6. d
2. c	7. d
3. b	8. a
4. d	9. b
5. b	10. d

Exercise 6—Case Study

Case Study 1

1. The tracheostomy tube is well visualized and placed. The tip is seen 3 to 4 cm above the carina.
2. In mobile imaging, it is common to do the image in the recumbent position. If there is a hemorrhage, it may be obscured. Tube placement is determined.
3. A pleural effusion or hemothorax could be obscured in the recumbent position; no fluid levels can be demonstrated.
4. A lateral decubitus; for fluid the affected side down, for air the affected side up.
5. There is a chest tube in the right pleural cavity.
6. The tube is to create a vacuum environment allowing a collapsed lung to reinflate or to remove excessive fluid in the pleural cavity.

Case Study 2

1. Not necessarily; it is difficult to see the tip of the catheter in this patient due to underexposure. It appears to be in the heart because it can be seen in the superior vena cava.
2. Those viewing the image should be able to see through the heart and mediastinum. The lung markings behind the heart should be visible and the outline of the spine should be visible through the mediastinum. If not, the image is considered underexposed. If an optimal kVp (100-130) is being used, the mAs needs to be increased.
3. The tracheostomy tube is well visualized and placed. The tip is seen 3 to 4 cm above the carina.
4. This would be a nasogastric (NG) tube. In this case, the patient has a tracheostomy and the oxygen is being supplemented at the ventilator. Always be sure to remove all movable tubing out of the image field to reduce artifacts.
5. The three lines represent the cardiac monitoring leads (EKG). They have been straightened and moved out of the image as much as possible. By disconnecting the lines, an alarm will sound if the patient is being closely monitored. The radiographer should not remove the

lines if the patient is in the intensive care unit and only when directed in other cases.

Case Study 3

1. Yes, the image contrast and density are balanced to demonstrate the tips of the leads.
2. Yes, the EKG lead is overlaying the superior pacer lead, which makes it difficult to distinguish. The radiographer needs to move the EKG leads to the side as much as possible.
3. In the atrium near the sinoatrial (SA) node
4. The inferior lead should be positioned at the apex of the right ventricle. It does appear in that region. A lateral projection would be required to demonstrate that the tip is directly posterior in the coronary sinus rather than in its proper position anterior in the right ventricle.

Self-Test

1.	d	6.	a
2.	c	7.	b
3.	c	8.	d
4.	b	9.	c
5.	d	10.	a